Acclaim for

The Ayurvedic Self-Care Handbook

"Dr. Kucera guides us in the practical application of rituals in the healing process of balancing the bodily humors and their circadian rhythms in our day-to-day lives. Applied in one's life, we can celebrate our lives through daily, seasonal, and healing rituals, thereby bringing more awareness to every aspect of our lives. A joyful, blissful book, it serves as a guideline to students and practitioners, unfolding inner healing and longevity."
—**Dr. Vasant Lad, BAM&S, MASc,** Ayurvedic physician, and author of *Ayurveda: The Science of Self-Healing* and the *Textbook of Ayurveda* series

"A wonderful book to upgrade your self-care rituals for more Ayurvedic magic in your life."—**Sahara Rose Ketabi,** best-selling author of *Eat Feel Fresh* and *Ayurveda (Idiot's Guides)*

"Kucera's expertise as a healer, both Ayurvedic practitioner and chiropractor, is abundantly evident in *The Ayurvedic Self-Care Handbook*, but what really shines through are her gifts as a *teacher*. This is the most accessible, logical, and practical yet never reductive book on Ayurveda I've ever read. It is now required reading for our Yoga Teacher Training programs!"—**Gina Caputo,** founder and director of the Colorado

D0873432

"A fresh, much-needed voice for Ayurvedic techniques of healing and balancing. *The Ayurvedic Self-Care Handbook* is an incredible manual for anyone who is ready to feel more balanced, energized, and radiant, while still showing up for everything that's on their (full) plate. I can't wait to share this with the women I work with."
—**Cassandra Bodzak,** author of *Eat With Intention*

"In our culture, where our traditions and rituals have been forgotten, *The Ayurvedic Self-Care Handbook* reminds us that our health, longevity, and happiness depend on our traditional circadian rituals."—**Dr. John Douillard, DC, CAP,** author of *The 3-Season Diet* and founder of LifeSpa.com

The Ayurvedic Self-Care Handbook

HOLISTIC HEALING RITUALS

for EVERY DAY AND SEASON

Sarah Kucera, DC, CAP

Foreword by Dr. Suhas Kshirsagar, BAMS, MD

THE EXPERIMENT

NEW YORK

The Experiment, LLC, 220 East 23rd Street, Suite 600, New York, NY 10010-4658
theexperimentpublishing.com

This book contains the opinions and ideas of its author. It is intended to provide helpful and informative material on the subjects addressed in the book. It is sold with the understanding that the author and publisher are not engaged in rendering medical, health, or any other kind of personal or professional services in the book. The author and publisher specifically disclaim all responsibility for any liability, loss, or risk—personal or otherwise—that is incurred as a consequence, directly or indirectly, of the use and application of any of the contents of this book.

Many of the designations used by manufacturers and sellers to distinguish their products are claimed as trademarks. Where those designations appear in this book and The Experiment was aware of a trademark claim, the designations have been capitalized.

The Experiment's books are available at special discounts when purchased in bulk for premiums and sales promotions as well as for fund-raising or educational use. For details, contact us at info@theexperimentpublishing.com.

Library of Congress Cataloging-in-Publication Data

Names: Kucera, Sarah, author.
Title: The ayurvedic self-care handbook : holistic healing rituals for every
   day and season / Sarah Kucera, DC, CAP ; foreword by Dr. Suhas Kshirsagar,
   BAMS, MD.
Description: New York, NY : Experiment, LLC, [2019] | Includes index.
Identifiers: LCCN 2018047856| ISBN 9781615195435 (cloth) | ISBN 9781615195442
   (ebook)
Subjects: LCSH: Medicine, Ayurvedic--Handbooks, manuals, etc. | Self-care,
   Health. | Holistic medicine.
Classification: LCC R605 .K757 2019 | DDC 615.5/38--dc23
LC record available at https://lccn.loc.gov/2018047856

ISBN 978-1-61519-543-5
Ebook ISBN 978-1-61519-544-2

Cover design by Sarah Smith | Text design by Sarah Schneider
Illustrations by Beth Bugler | Author photograph by Suzanne Corum-Rich

Manufactured in China
First printing April 2019
10 9 8 7 6 5 4 3 2 1

*This book is dedicated to all of my patients and students.
Whether it was one class or appointment, or many
throughout the years, you have trusted me to be your guide.
As I have been your teacher, you have also been mine.
I am so thankful for you.*

Table of Contents

by Dr. Suhas Kshirsagar

he Ayurvedic Self-Care Handbook is a perfect template to take control of your health and well-being. All the latest medical research converges upon evidence that a plant-based diet, sleep, exercise, meditation, and effective stress management are the keys for everyday health. There is no better template than Ayurvedic medicine to integrate these modalities. In fact, Ayurveda is the art and science of longevity.

We are at a crossroads in medicine where we need to regain our understanding of the true meaning of prevention, which means we must participate in our own health and make responsible choices. All the ancient cultures understood the importance of self-care rituals that were perfectly aligned with the phases of moon, changing seasons, festivals, and community living. Healthy living was a way of life, and social well-being was based upon sustainable living.

The latest science of chronobiology supports this ancient wisdom, clearly revealing that time is embedded in our genes. The timing of eating, sleep, and exercise are all very important to how we digest the world around us (not just food), which translates into our physical, emotional, and spiritual health. This emerging Western research is exciting, but it also validates the ancient Ayurvedic principles of daily, nightly, and seasonal routines for people in various phases of life, which I've explored throughout my work and writings.

The book in your hands is paramount for promoting self-love and self-responsibility in today's modern age. Sarah Kucera is a good friend and colleague who is at the forefront of sharing these concepts with her clients and students alike. A chiropractor by training, she is combining this science of the body with her deeply intuitive yogic and Ayurvedic perspectives, to identify and correct the root imbalance causing disease, and to empower people in owning their health. Ayurveda and yoga are sister sciences that empower us to lead a spiritual life free from diseases. Their prescriptions are not quite what most of us are used to, however; this ancient system's medicine involves simple forms of self-care—such as daily oil massage, morning walks, herbal teas, spices, and healing foods—all of which not only prevent the imbalances that cause disease, but also improve the overall quality and quantity of our lives.

Although self-care is growing in popularity, it's largely been a completely foreign concept in the West. As industry and the economy advance, we have become conditioned to yearn, struggle, and strive for more, and to continuously work hard. Many individuals in the workforce—especially millennials—fear being away from the office, forgetting about vacations and paid time off. The majority of my patients struggle with these concerns, battling disappointment, burnout, and depression that affects their work and personal lives. Needless to say, this puts tremendous pressure on their families and all the relationships they engage in, perpetuating unhealthy work-life balance and the neglect of self-care. We cannot love others if we don't love ourselves first.

Everyone shares a natural desire to be happy—the purpose of life itself is simply the expansion of happiness. Most people, however, seek happiness from external sources. At a certain point, we learn that happiness is a state of being rather than something that is acquired. You cannot choose what you experience in everyday life, whether a traffic jam or a rainbow. But you can choose to cultivate an attitude of looking at the brighter side of things, and not to ingest the toxicity of any experience. This practice alone will set up the conditions for a truly sattvic—or balanced and joyful—state; a state that relies on self-love as the source of happiness.

Self-love can be defined as the act of valuing one's own happiness and well-being. It is a kind of acceptance, or unconditional support and caring. And it is at the core of compassion for self-healing. It requires commitment to oneself, as well as willingness to identify and to meet personal needs, to allow non-judgmental thinking, and to view the self as essentially worthy, good, valuable, and deserving of health and happiness. All from deep within ourselves, not the outside.

As Sarah clearly and thoroughly outlines in this heartfelt book, the easiest way to do this according to Ayurvedic philosophy is through aligning with nature. Natural biorhythms are constantly affecting our mind and body, and so conscious efforts to follow daily as well as seasonal routines will help us prevent imbalance. Building from there, if you can balance your day, you will soon be able to balance your thoughts and listen to your body. And with that, you can change your life.

The real reason for self-care and self-love, however, isn't as selfish as it may sound. We are trying to discover balance for greater harmony inside and outside ourselves. When we are healthy—physically, mentally, and emotionally—our state of well-being spills out to everyone in our lives. As we learn self-acceptance, self-forgiveness, and self-compassion, we become more empathetic and tolerant of humanity. The way we treat ourselves also sends a powerful message to our friends, family, and even the general population, about how we accept being treated. If we are consistently putting ourselves last, we should not be surprised when others do the same—and yet, when others become dismissive and disrespectful, we are hurt profoundly, taking it personally, feeling like a victim in the system that we perpetuate by our own unconscious behavior.

Sarah does a phenomenal job outlining many different forms of self-love, providing the most comprehensive guide for well-being. Grounded in her own experience, she has made it her personal mission to share the necessity of self-love and self-care as a cornerstone of happiness and, indeed, optimum health. Whether you incorporate just one of the rituals in these pages, or find yourself rescheduling your entire life, by picking up this book you're already on your way to a more balanced, aligned, and awake version of yourself—and to learning to love and care for yourself in a new, radiant light.

Dr. Suhas Kshirsagar, BAMS, MD (Ayurveda), is a world-renowned Ayurvedic physician and educator from India, and the director of the Ayurvedic Healing and Integrative Wellness Clinic in northern California. He is the author of *The Hot Belly Diet* and *Change Your Schedule, Change Your Life.*

The Nature of Medicine

Whenever I'm struggling with feeling less than my best, I think back to when I was healthiest and happiest—an exercise I recommend we all do on occasion. Without hesitation my mind goes back to my childhood, around age nine to be precise. I grew up in small-town Iowa, where I ate home-cooked meals bursting with the flavors of my mother's garden or my grandparents' farm; I had the freedom to fearlessly play outside, biking in the summer and sledding in the winter; my and my older sister's days followed a solid routine that was undoubtedly shaped by my mom's desire to raise healthy and happy children. After all, that was how she was raised herself. As one of five children growing up in a small farmhouse, she was given a schedule of daily chores, but also an abundance of nurturing from her own mother. Her days had predictability, and so mine did, too. I can remember not only how my nine-year-old days opened and closed, but also the feeling of safety my routine provided.

It's possible my current passion for routine and rituals—a passion I've built my career on, as an Ayurvedic practitioner and in other ways—is subconsciously rooted in experiencing such comfort and security as a child, not yet knowing the responsibilities adulthood would bring. Even as I grew older and moved away from the family farm and table, I always felt my truest self when my life was guided by nature and the rituals that accompany it. Nature is methodical and gives us all the important cues we need for health and balance: when to rise and when to sleep, when to eat and when to move. The daily activities, meals, and decorations cued by the changes in season were what kept my family healthy and created a warmth in our home. They were the opposite of rigid and monotonous, like my current "to-dos" can feel.

As we are sentient beings, living in line with nature should be instinctual, but our modern life has pulled us away from this. In my early twenties, caught up in my own desires to achieve, I found myself looking for ways to make life convenient, seeking out the most up-to-date technology and devices, and often prioritizing work over self-care. But as I began to learn more about Ayurveda, I realized I had become disconnected from the ways my small-town youth kept me aligned with nature. I was no longer paying attention to my intuition.

For over 5,000 years, Ayurveda has taught that people exist on a continuum with nature, and that we should honor this connection through the foods we eat, the way we conduct our day, and by fully taking in our changing environment through our senses. Nature is cyclical, and when our lives flow in sync with it, we feel well. When life—and the distractions of technology, work, stress, etc.—causes us to veer off track, we experience imbalance, only to leave us desperate and searching for a way to get back in line.

We are lucky in that our earliest ancestors evolved immersed in nature instead of in their devices. They observed the fluctuations of the twenty-four-hour clock and seasonal cycles in both our internal and external environments, developing an understanding that illness arises when we go against nature or our own internal wisdom. When we feel tired but don't sleep, we become more susceptible to common colds and flus because we've lowered our immunity; similarly, we are more likely to develop unhealthy digestive conditions when we eat food that has been engineered, lacks natural nourishment, or is grown out of season. As Ayurvedic practitioners observed these propensities for sicknesses, the recommendations for daily, nightly, and seasonal routines were born—including the foundational eating and sleeping patterns that remained mainstays in generations as recent as our grandparents.

Unlike many others, I didn't discover Ayurveda and learn about the regimen for self-care at a time when I needed recalibrating. Rather, I was attracted to it as a potential bridge between my education as both a chiropractor and a yoga teacher since Ayurveda is known as yoga's "sister science," the study of the body that complements yoga's study of the mind. There was beauty in the idea that our kitchens could become our pharmacies, and in how food possesses qualities beyond carbohydrates, fats, and proteins, making diet both medicinal and customizable to one's constitution. These concepts would give me the ability to treat conditions outside of the musculoskeletal complaints I was most often addressing in my chiropractic practice, in addition to taking my own health to the next level.

As I began to see patients under the title of an Ayurvedic practitioner, diet and herbal therapies were my favorite things to discuss and the top interest of those coming to see me. Even though routine had been so paramount in my health growing up and in my life at the time, I was putting emphasis on the *what* of my patients' routines instead of the *how*. And while it seems as if many people are drawn to alternative medicines such as Ayurveda, Chinese medicine, homeopathy, or naturopathy because supplements and herbs are used instead of Western prescription medications, I found myself questioning if this was what natural medicine was all about. I suddenly couldn't ignore that the most effective thing about Ayurveda wasn't the doshic-specific diet or the adaptogenic herbs, but rather the following of daily and seasonal self-care rituals, which Ayurveda has stood by for thousands of years. It occurred to me that Ayurveda isn't a "natural" medicine because of its absence of pharmaceuticals, but because the medicine is nature itself.

At the same time, I personally was on the verge of burnout. Living out of sync with Ayurveda's recommended routines, I filled my free time with work to meet the demands of being a small business owner; on top of that, my work was in offering care to others, and so like many in these "helper" professions, my inclination was always to give, leaving little freedom for leisure or even the most basic rituals that I knew would set a foundation for my day. The only constant was a harried and unsettled sensation in my body and mind. Despite being a minimalist and tidy person, I'd have piles of clean laundry on my floor for days or weeks because I didn't have the energy to put them away. I love learning activities, such as watching documentaries and listening to TED Talks, but I only had time to zone out to Netflix when I came home at night. I prefer to cook my meals, but I had carryout several times a week because going to the store to buy food and then prepare it was a daunting task. All in all, I didn't feel like myself.

Believing it didn't have to be that way, I recruited nature—my lifelong ally—to change. I set morning and evening rituals in accordance with my needs and circumstances. I embraced my internal environment with meditation and periodic breaks during my day so that I could take inventory of how I was feeling mentally, physically, and emotionally. I acclimated myself to my external environment by spending more time outdoors, even as the seasonal temperatures in my home of Kansas City, Missouri, vacillated between extreme summer heat and extreme winter cold. I became dedicated to connecting with nature and its cycles by taking a walk in the fresh air every morning and committing to sleeping and eating at the same time each day. I realized that the independent work that was burning me out also allowed me to set my own schedule—no one was stopping me from eating lunch at the same time every day except me. These practices from Ayurveda and my healthy upbringing created a container for my life.

Suddenly, I started to feel like my nine-year-old self in my adult body. I may not have been playing tag out in a field or helping my mother clean vegetables from the garden for dinner, but my health flourished. A reflection of my new commitments to rituals, routines, and aligning myself with nature, I felt well *and* good.

I began emphasizing Ayurveda's routines in my patients' treatment plans and they'd arrive to their follow-up visits looking brighter and happier, and reporting an improvement in their sleep, digestion, and energy. This approach was not only reducing their symptoms, but also creating a sound foundation for better health.

My hope in this book is to illuminate for you a new possibility for health through simple rituals, sensible changes, and the use of nature as your ally. Acting as your trail guide, I draw upon ancient and modern medicines alike, my personal experience, and the ways my patients have used routine to heal digestive issues, skin conditions, hormonal imbalances, sleep disorders, and fatigue. You'll find Ayurveda's most foundational principles outlined, including the five elements, the three constitutions (*doshas*), and the specific qualities used to describe them. You'll learn how nature and the twenty-four-hour clock dictate our physiology from the perspective of both Ayurveda and circadian medicine. We'll discuss the importance of rituals and those practices that Ayurveda recommends we do on a daily and seasonal basis to maintain health, while also identifying how your strengths and vulnerabilities can impact your success. For those times you encounter obstacles or aversions, there are tips for troubleshooting; and for the times that you aren't feeling well, there are suggestions for a variety of self-care rituals and practices to nurse yourself back to health.

As you learn about the richly intuitive system of Ayurveda, you'll deepen your understanding about yourself. In this way, you'll find Ayurveda to be like a friend of many years who simply "gets you." Within both yogic and Ayurvedic philosophies, there is a concept called svadhyaya, which means "self-study." Because we can really only find true health when we know our true self, self-study questions are included throughout as well as sample journaling prompts for helping you maintain your rituals. Together, these exercises will help you become more aware of your personal habits, patterns, and thought processes, and use that awareness to make better choices for how you want to feel.

Rituals can give form to our lives by creating space for the self-care that is necessary to support those goals. My hope is that this book will inspire you to go for more walks outside, wake up with the sun, and learn what it means to eat seasonal food based on where you live. I wish for it to be the infrastructure to an energetic life spent doing the things you love with the people you care about most. These pages hold the plan for you to become the best version of yourself—the self uniquely designed by nature to not only live and feel well, but grow, share, and thrive.

PART 1

Consistent, Cyclical, Meaningful

CHAPTER 1

Ayurveda

The Embodiment of Nature

yurveda (from *ayur* meaning "life," and *veda* meaning "knowledge" or "science of") is a system of healing from India that uses nature as medicine, in a preventive and curative sense. It uses food, spices, herbal therapies, bodywork, and lifestyle changes to create the conditions of optimal health. It's all-encompassing, in that it aims to use your personal story to create a specialized path for healing. It's quite possible that the most comforting thing Ayurveda has to offer is its ability to understand you as you are, not some hypothetical "you" from a textbook. It appreciates your uniqueness and knows how to treat you as an individual. It offers explanations for things you've always known about yourself but haven't been able to articulate, implement, or accept.

This adeptness in knowing and interpreting what makes you tick isn't a magical or psychic phenomenon. Living by Ayurveda doesn't require converting to a religion, practicing any mystical ceremonies, or even practicing yoga. It is science and arises from nature—both the observation of our external environment and the understanding that we are not separate from it. This is also the most foundational principle in Ayurveda, known as the *macrocosm microcosm continuum theory*. Simply put, the theory states that we (the microcosm) are a reflection of the universe (the macrocosm), and as such everything that exists outside of us also exists within us. This means that any shift in nature causes us to change, and that our actions can also strongly impact nature.

With our universe being as vast as it is, the continuum theory can be tough to grasp at first, even a bit scary. It's one thing to know your actions affect you alone, but to have them affect other people—even the planet—is something else entirely. Yet as we divide nature into smaller components, things seem more manageable. When we accept nature's elements and understand the roles they play, we can lessen our desire to be in control of how we feel. We become responsive to our surroundings rather than resistant.

Elements, or Bhutas

When you attempt to live in harmony with nature, you aren't connecting with only one large entity, but rather something made up of several smaller parts. Ayurveda defines nature as being comprised of five elements, or *bhutas*: ether (or space), air, fire, water, and earth. They are present in everything, including us, and we need all of these things to survive. We need space to expand, air to breathe, the sun to transform or grow, water to hydrate, and the earth to nourish. And while the concept of everything being made of the same elements could be suggestive of everyone looking, thinking, and acting the same, the opposite is true. The elements are expressed differently and in varying degrees in each of us, making each thing and being unique. You can easily see this in Earth's weather, as we have sunny days with more fire, windy days with more air, and rainy or humid days that are full of water.

This is observed in our food, too: Root vegetables that grow in the ground carry a greater expression of earth, whereas you can feel the fire in spicy foods like peppers. And in ourselves and other human beings, the rule of elements is just as present. You've certainly encountered people you'd describe as "spacey," others who are "hot-headed," and some who are "grounded." There are those whose mind will change with the wind and others who are more like rocks and unwilling to budge. When someone has more earth expressed in their physical body, they will be taller or have bigger muscles or bones, compared to the presence

SELF-STUDY

Begin to understand how the elements are represented in you. What are the ways you express ether, air, fire, water, and earth in your mind and emotions? Do you notice a greater or lesser expression of certain elements in your physical body? Do you feel more connected to one specific element?

of air, which produces a more delicate frame and features. Stop to look and you'll see—the five elements are found in everyone and everywhere.

Qualities, or Gunas

Now that you have a grasp on the concept of elements, let's explore another principle that makes the system of Ayurveda more relatable: the *gunas*. The gunas are attributes or qualities that are used to describe the elements and are paired in opposites. There are ten pairs, with each descriptor in the pair being at one end of a continuum: dry/oily, light/heavy, mobile/static, rough/smooth, cold/hot, clear/cloudy, hard/soft, liquid/dense, sharp/dull, subtle/gross. Each element carries its own combination of properties—for example; air is dry, light, and mobile, but earth is oily, heavy, and static. (See Table 1, page 20.)

Since the elements are found everywhere and in everyone, these words are used to describe all things, ranging from the foods we eat and the experiences we have to the symptoms we feel. Did you have a heavy or a light lunch today? Was it a rough day at work, or did things go smoothly? Are you thinking clearly or are your thoughts clouded? Is your skin as dry as your humor? Are you sharp-minded or do you have a sharp tongue? There are so many ways that we use these qualifiers in daily life, but we rarely pause to consider that they are more than just semantics.

The concept of gunas is as important as it is basic, and quite possibly the most empowering concept in Ayurveda. When you can understand where you inherently lie on each of these continuums and what descriptors your imbalances have in common, you hold the key to your own healing. As you'll learn later, qualities can accumulate and too much of one thing will leave you feeling unwell. Though it almost sounds too simplistic or easy to be true, you feel better by incorporating the opposite quality on the continuum into your life.

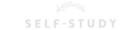

SELF-STUDY

Looking at the twenty gunas, which five most closely relate to health conditions you currently or commonly experience?

The Three Constitutions, or Doshas

Nature, the elements, and their descriptors are all neatly packaged into Ayurvedic constitutions called *doshas*. The doshas give a concise picture of how nature is represented in us, while simultaneously giving an explanation of how our physiology works, and providing meaning to why each of us has our own specific strengths, weaknesses, and needs. There are three doshas—*vata, pitta,* and *kapha*—and each is composed of two of the five elements. But just as all of the elements exist within us, all of the doshas are within us, too. Each is responsible for governing different tissues, organs, and functions of the body; so, similar to how we couldn't live without air or water, we couldn't live without having each constitution present.

Your unique expression of your constitution explains everything about you, from your bone structure to the color of your eyes to the texture of your hair. It tells about the ways your physical characteristics and personal interests are actually related, and the way you react to stress, or the illnesses you most frequently experience. As you read on to learn about each dosha, begin to think of the aspects of each you see in yourself and which resonates with you most, keeping in mind all are a part of you.

Vata

The **vata dosha** is made of ether and air, and has the qualities of light, subtle, dry, rough, hard, clear, cold, and mobile. Vata governs our nervous system, hearing, elimination, and all movement in the body, including the movement at our joints and the circulation of blood and lymph (fluid that's a part of your immune system and contains white blood cells and lymphocytes). In our physical traits, vata appears as coarse or curly hair, a small or petite frame, lean or sinewy muscles, and delicate facial features, like thin lips, small eyes, or small teeth. Those with a higher proportion of vata tend to get cold easily and frequently experience dryness, such as in their skin or eyes. In psychological traits, the combination of ether and air enables creative and spontaneous sides, but this blend can also heighten emotions like fear, indecisiveness, or worry. Vatas will gravitate toward such career paths as artists, creators, or jobs that require more movement than sitting. They can love to travel, be known as social butterflies, or generally enjoy change.

Pitta

Fire and water make up the **pitta dosha**, which is described as light, sharp, hot, liquid, and dry or oily. It keeps watch over our ability to transform and governs our hormones, enzymes, digestion, blood, skin, and eyes. Physically this constitution has an average-size stature and a sharpness in their facial features, such as a well-defined jawline, pointy nose, or piercing blue or green eyes. Their hair is commonly fine or thin, and is often blond, red, or early to go gray. As for the mind, pittas are known to be the thinkers, problem solvers, goal setters, and leaders. Those with this dosha have a passion that makes them want to do their best, and even the competitiveness to do better than others. But this intensity can also cause them to become frustrated, angry, or irritable more easily that the other doshas. Their focus on achievement means they seek out influential roles in society or careers that require higher education, which is why doctors, lawyers, politicians, and CEOs are often pitta-predominant.

Kapha

The **kapha dosha** is a combination of water and earth, giving it adequate properties for protection and growth within the body. It's described as heavy, dense, static, dull, gross, smooth, soft, cloudy, and warm or cool. In our physiology, it's in charge of our respiratory system, heart, brain, immunity, mucous membranes, cartilage, and synovial fluid. You'd be right to guess this support-ive nature means kaphas will have the sturdiest structure, with bigger bones and bulkier muscles. These qualities also provide them with thick and lustrous hair, milky skin, big, compassionate eyes, and full lips. They appreciate stability more than change, and are non-confrontational people who are like peacemakers, interested in everyone around them being happy. While these stable qualities are desirable, they can also create a heaviness that leads toward depression, sluggishness, or feeling stuck. As such steadfast beings, kaphas are usually in nurturing and supportive roles in our society. Many with a lot of kapha in their constitution choose to become caregivers, teachers, nurses, or social workers.

Though all doshas are present within all of us, and you will relate to each one to some extent, we are each likely to have one or two that are more prevalent. This is called your *prakruti*, or your inherent constitution, which is said to be determined upon conception. The time, place, and context under which you were conceived, along with your parents' health at the time, were all crucial in creating your makeup.

Your dosha or constitution never changes. Your tendencies and vulnerabilities as a child are the same ones you deal with now. What does change is whether or not you are living within a balance of your true self, surfing life's waves and managing small fluctuations. In this case, balance doesn't mean equal amounts of each dosha, but rather the maintenance of your personal dosha recipe. So when you set out to achieve "perfect health" according to Ayurveda, you are really aiming to keep the proportion of doshas determining your constitution intact, as *your* nature made them.

There is great value in knowing your dosha or constitution. However, what is most useful is being able to recognize how a dosha can either support you, or accumulate and block you. While there is an abundance of dosha quizzes online and in books to help you determine your constitution, I have intentionally omitted one from this book. It's too easy to take a quiz, which may not be reliable, and even easier to allow it to become your identity in a rigid and limiting way. Instead of using your budding knowledge of how you feel to label or categorize yourself, use it to understand more about you in each moment: about your physiology, the reasons you excel at certain things, and how you make decisions each day. Then, in time, you can meet with an Ayurvedic practitioner, who can help you more accurately assess your constitution.

SELF-STUDY

It's important to understand how each dosha is represented and expressed uniquely in you, in your thoughts, actions, emotions, and even physical characteristics. For each dosha in the table, create a list of the corresponding qualities that apply to you. Use your new Ayurvedic lenses to take note of your daily activities and if they are activities that would interest a vata, pitta, or kapha. Without becoming attached to one, which do you identify with most?

Table 1. Dosha Overview

DOSHA	ELEMENTS	QUALITIES	ASSOCIATED FUNCTIONS + TISSUES	QUALITIES OF HEALTHY CONSTITUTION	SIGNS OF IMBALANCE
Vata	Ether + Air	Light, mobile, clear, subtle, dry, rough, hard, cold	All movement, circulation, joints, nervous system, hearing, speaking, elimination, colon	Creativity, spontaneity, social butterfly, full of ideas	Anxiety, worry, fear, insomnia, dry skin, constipation, cold hands and feet, restlessness, nerve pain, weight gain in hips and thighs, depletion, emaciation, inability to concentrate
Pitta	Fire + Water	Light, sharp, oily or dry, hot, liquid	Blood, eyes, skin, hormones, enzymes, digestion, emotional heart, small intestine, liver	Confident, natural leader, sharp intellect	Anger, frustration, judgment, hyperacidity, weight gain in abdomen, loose or soft bowel movements, blood in stool, burnout, hypertension, rashes or inflammatory skin conditions
Kapha	Water + Earth	Heavy, static, dense, oily, smooth, soft, dull, cloudy, gross, warm or cool	Lungs, brain, adipose, synovial fluid, cartilage, mucosal linings, immune system, lymph, heart, stomach	Compassionate, nurturing, desire to help and provide care, stable	Depression, weight gain in torso or chest, swelling, fluid retention, sluggish digestion, mucus in stool, productive cough, high cholesterol, elevated blood sugar, oily skin

Like Increases Like:
How We Experience Imbalance

It's important that we appease our constitution, to feed the things that we love and to foster our strengths and talents, but when we take things to the extreme or fail to counter with the opposing qualities, we can experience imbalance. Imbalance comes from an influx—either slow and steady, or sudden and abrupt—of a quality, element, or dosha, and is called *vikruti.* Though this can occur from a dosha being subdued or depleted, it is most often discussed as an accumulation or increase. For example, if on one of the coldest days of winter you decided to eat your lunch of a raw salad outside and wash it down with an iced beverage, the excessive cold would start to make you feel uncomfortable. You might be able to mentally override this or eventually feel better after spending time in the air of your artificially heated home, but if you had to sustain this for many hours or for many days, the level of discomfort would begin to increase and be more challenging to resolve, no matter how much you enjoy salads or the winter. Without opposing heating qualities to level things out, the cold will continue to rise and to manifest as symptoms, increasing their severity in time. This is the principle of accumulation, or "like increases like," which is at the heart of every ailment we have, physical, emotional, and psychological.

No matter what your overall constitution is, you can have an imbalance in any dosha (or quality or element); however, you are more susceptible to the dosha that is already highest in you. Picture it like this: If you have three buckets of water and two of them are only one-third full while the other is filled to the brim, any of them could overflow if you were to add enough water, but the one that is nearest full would overflow the quickest. The doshas are exactly the same. Someone who typically has oily skin (kapha) can still experience dry skin (vata) if they eat an excessive amount of drying foods or are exposed to dry air and wind, but it would take more for them to get to that point than someone who naturally has dry skin in the first place.

Similarly, our dosha also gives insight as to *where* in our body we might have these imbalances. Remember how each dosha governs certain tissues? You are more likely to have imbalances manifest in the organs that your primary constitution governs. For example, given the right scenario, a vata person could certainly experience a hormonal imbalance, but because pitta governs hormones, the pitta person is typically more readily affected in this way, whereas a vata-predominant person is more likely to first experience problems with their nervous system, joints, or colon.

These principles of imbalance are part of what makes Ayurveda an accessible system, but understandably, it can be difficult to comprehend at first. Use Table 1 on page 20 as a guide for getting to know more about how each dosha relates to you and the symptoms you experience. And above all, become an observer of how different foods, activities, and even people make you feel.

CHAPTER 2

Identifying a Need for Change

Your Current Health Status and
the Baseline for Optimal Health

You are happiest and healthiest when you are being you. We polish our innate skills and talents until they shine like precious gems, which makes it easy to tell when we're not being given the chance to shine. If you're a creative and you're denied the outlet to create, you'll feel like you're suffocating. If you're a leader and learner, but lack an environment that fosters a sense of autonomy or progress, you'll feel frustrated and out of control. If you're a caregiver with a compassionate heart, you'll feel empty if you're unable to serve others.

This doesn't mean, however, that we should only strive to be in our best state all the time. Even the most perfect gems have flaws, and since we may never entirely rub out our less desirable traits and habits, we learn how to accept and manage them as part of our unique constitution. This isn't the same as admitting defeat or complacency, or accepting we're not enough; instead, it is learning to release expectation and give ourselves a break.

The occasional rut is to be epected, but when we continually don't feel our best, it's time to make a shift. Recognizing a need for change isn't always easy. We can be stuck in our own cycles, aware that compliance with our external environment is beneficial, but unaware that we are doing the wrong things to stay balanced. As the saying goes, if you keep doing what you have always done, you'll keep getting what you have always gotten. And likely, if you're reading this book, you have an innate desire to get something else out of your life.

Samskara is a Sanskrit word that describes the mental impression created by our experiences. When we repeat actions throughout our days and lives, these samskaras create "grooves." They can

---

SELF-STUDY

Think about times in your life when you felt happiest and "in the groove." Then, reflect on your daily patterns/grooves, and how they compare to that time. Are there things you do every day to feel good? What happens if you don't do them? Is there anything you aren't doing every day or week that you know would make you feel better? Are there things that make you feel bad?

be positive grooves, such as responding selflessly when witnessing someone in need; but they can also be negative, and feel more like a rut or obstacle to self-evolution. If you can identify these samskaras, and you're willing to recognize areas for improvement, you can break the cycle and forge new, more natural grooves.

It's time to sit down for some one-on-one time with yourself to see if you've been treading in one of these grooves and if you could benefit from a lifestyle shake-up. The list of questions to ask when determining such could be quite long, so let's start with the more common and recognizable concerns. The questions below address the issues that I've seen most often with the patients in my clinical practice. These are also aligned with what Ayurveda uses as a baseline for health: small imbalances that you may not typically consider symptomatic, that may almost feel "natural," but are really samskaras and cause enough for concern. As you consider these yes-or-no questions, be sure you are in a quiet place with a clear mind, and no pending to-dos awaiting your attention, so you can answer honestly.

- Do you feel like you are doing all the right things to stay healthy, but still seem to feel unwell?
- Is your energy consistently low or less than what you need to do the things you want to do in life? Likewise, does your energy fluctuate in significant ways day-to-day, or season-to-season?
- Are you waking up during the night or having difficulty falling asleep?

- Do you experience brain fog, difficulty remembering, or feel like you've lost your mental sharpness?
- Is your digestion offtrack? How?
- Does your skin (face and body) lack luster, or have blemishes, rashes, or dryness/oiliness?
- Would you describe yourself as anxious, burned out, depressed, or unhappy? Does your mood impact your relationships?
- Are you missing out on the things in life that feed your soul?

Would it be a spoiler to say that answering "yes" to any of these suggests you need a change? This doesn't come with the implication that you should try harder to fix things, but rather, it implies that you should stop and evaluate if things could be different. So many times we resign ourselves to the idea that what we are experiencing is normal: a part of aging, or a fleeting symptom that will take care of itself in time. But in many cases, this isn't true. Likewise, we can overlook underlying causes when we don't stop to check in, and the little things start to add up—going back to the theory of accumulation. You may not be slowing down enough to notice the smaller ways your routine, or lack thereof, is impacting you right now, but if you're going against nature, a bigger manifestation will eventually stop you in your tracks.

For example, Ayurveda has a rule for the temperature at which one should consume liquids that is applicable to all constitutions. It's said that if we drink cold or iced drinks, we run the risk of putting out our digestive fire and reducing our ability to process what we consume. If having iced water with your meal was an isolated instance, it could wreak havoc on your digestion for that day. But if you continue to consume iced drinks every day or several times every day, the frequency, duration, and degree of the effects would increase. A condition becomes more extensive and difficult to treat the longer the insult to your body continues. This is also seen in the case of some food sensitivities. When you eat a certain food every day, either out of pleasure or interest in receiving its health benefits, but your digestion isn't doing well at breaking it down and eliminating it, at some point your body will give you the sign to not consume any more. For some, this is as basic as the taste not being as satisfying as it once was, but for others it could cause indigestion or skin irritations. This shouldn't make you label the food as "good" or "bad"; just interpret this as information from your body that it's time for a change—and an opportunity to try something new!

It's also vital that your daily actions align with your overall values. Rituals encourage impeccable mental hygiene, not only physical balance. If you disregard how a few minutes in the morning and evening can shift your mindset and keep you connected to your greater intentions for life, you risk feeling stuck, overwhelmed, and disappointed.

SELF-STUDY

Do you participate in things regularly about which you feel guilt or regret afterward? Are there things you do regularly that get in the way of actualizing your ideal life? What are these things and why have they become a part of your routine?

A revamped routine could allow you to be content while still evolving, thus avoiding complacency or stagnation. Your new or altered routine should incorporate the things that you intuitively know make you feel like your truest self. If that includes an occasional indulgence in cookies or French fries that is too infrequent to negatively impact your health, by all means eat them! But remember that we can react negatively to anything in abundance.

This is why you need to be clear about your intentions before you start building new rituals into your day. If your dream life isn't the one you're living now, make note of the things you want to be different. Be detailed as possible about your personal and professional goals. Give yourself gentle reminders and mini steps to reach toward what you are trying to achieve. Soon you'll see how improving one aspect of your life improves others, as tripping one cycle can help all rhythms regain synchronicity.

Establish Your Baseline

It can be difficult to believe that an idea as simple as committing to daily rituals could solve complex or chronic health problems. Just like imbalances don't (always) happen overnight, changes don't always happen quickly. So when making an intentional change, it's important not only to document your starting point, but also to understand what you should be looking for as indicators of a need for better health. Your digestion, sleep, vibrancy of your skin, physical energy, and mental energy are the first things to observe on your quest to feel your best. Maybe you only feel off in a small way and it's easy to recover, like when a spicy meal disrupts your digestion for one day or you're kept awake for one night by thoughts of a stressful day or sick loved one. These are the smaller imbalances that occur simply from the flux of life. But you should document anything that has been more of a constant, which in general means it has been present for more than one to two weeks. For example, when you have constipation or loose stool for seven days in a row, or you haven't gotten an uninterrupted night of sleep in two weeks, this is a sign that something bigger is happening. If other symptoms haven't appeared yet, they will soon. Following Ayurveda's main diagnostic principles below, however, can help you prevent an underlying imbalance from getting worse.

Digestion

The health of your digestion is a measure of how well you are processing what you take in, and how well you are eliminating it. This is important for making sure you receive the proper nutrients and fuel, and that waste, or what you don't need, is efficiently being removed. In Ayurveda, digestion is referred to as a fire, called *agni*. Strong agni equates to good health. Healthy elimination is having a bowel movement every day, one to two times per day. Ayurveda says that our ideal bowel movement happens first thing in the morning and looks like an overly ripe banana still in its peel in its size, shape, consistency, and brown color. Though feelings like bloating, burping, gas, hyperacidity, and stomach pains are common, know they aren't normal or healthy. Additionally, you should never really feel different after you eat. If a meal relieves feelings of intense hunger, then you've waited too long to eat. When you feel tired after eating, you either didn't eat the right things to nourish yourself, your eating times were too close to one another, or your digestion is sluggish. Your rituals around eating can positively impact these things.

Sleep

A proper night of sleep is essential for the restoration of our body and mind. When we were children, bedtime rituals were key, and our parents did everything they could to get us to sleep through the night. But everyone at any age deserves, and needs, a full night's sleep. Remember this as you are evaluating your current baseline. Unless disrupted sleep is caused by an outside interruption, such as a co-sleeper, child, or pet, it isn't normal. You should fall asleep within ten minutes of going to bed and stay asleep until your alarm goes off the next morning.

Skin

Your skin is the biggest organ of your body, and in Ayurveda, there is a strong relationship between our liver and blood health and the health of our skin. It's a common myth that we release toxins through our skin, yet its health does reflect what is happening on the inside. Often imbalances from our sleep, digestion, and stress level will show up as minor changes in our skin, such as dryness, redness, or acne, before a more advanced health condition occurs. A breakout from time to time or an occasional need to use more oils or lotions to keep your skin hydrated will go along with the ebb and flow of diet, lifestyle, and weather and shouldn't have you worried. However, as a general guideline, your skin (all over your body, not just on your face) should have an even tone, be clear of blemishes, feel naturally hydrated, and have a healthy elasticity that feels plump instead of papery. Everyone, not just pregnant women, should be told they look—and should feel—like they're "glowing" on the outside, as a reflection of true inner health. Get a good look at that mug prior to starting your rituals so you can appreciate the new picture of wellness you see in the mirror once the right rituals for you are in place.

Physical Energy

Low energy is among the top complaints of my patients, whether it is primary or secondary to other symptoms. It's right for them to be concerned, as not having enough energy to do the things you enjoy, let alone enough to get through your workday, is a sign that you're not taking enough time for rest, or that you aren't being properly fueled. Of course, we want to have as much energy as possible, but start by evaluating if your energy is consistent or fluctuates throughout the day. It's ideal for it to be steady and at a level that we feel we can comfortably complete desired tasks. We have a natural decrease around 7 or 8 PM, but until then you shouldn't feel listless or restless. In your best state of health, you should wake with energy that is sustained throughout the day, without feeling weak, hyper, or like you are looking forward to your next opportunity to sleep. Often times people say that they aren't tired during the day, but that they fall asleep if they sit down to watch a movie or immediately as their head hits the pillow. This typically means they don't stop to assess their energy, and they push through low points only to crash whenever they stop to sit.

Mental or Emotional Energy

The energy of our physical body and of our mind are as inter-related as they are independent. Mental or emotional energy is measured by your memory, your clarity of mind, the stability of your mood, and how you react to stress. And just as we'd like to be physically energized throughout the day, it's also necessary that we have enough mental energy to process thoughts, have intelligent discussions, and make sound decisions. You should be able to think and communicate without it feeling like there is strain or effort. While making decisions may not be your forte, it shouldn't be a process that generates overwhelming fear or worry. And while we are all entitled to a bad day, our reactions and responses to stress should be proportionate to the stressors. Trust that it *is* possible to feel mentally energized every day, and that there can be quick recovery from your simple emotional fluctuations.

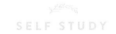

SELF STUDY

Using the list of parameters above, take some time to journal about how you've felt over the last two weeks in each category, or start now and record it for the next two weeks. What patterns have emerged?

CHAPTER 3

It's a Matter of Time

Learning the Ayurvedic and Circadian Clocks

One of the only things we know for certain is that the sun will rise and set every day. No matter the decisions we make in our own personal lives, Mother Nature is always making the grandest gesture of all. Through light alone, she tells the trees when to bear fruit and the flowers when to blossom. She organizes the patterns of our weather and the change of our seasons. Yet she is also the conductor of so much more than that.

It's great fortune that we have an industrialized world that has made it easier for us to access food and medicine. But with this gain, we have also lost. The 2010 census showed a whopping 80.7 percent of the U.S. population lived in urban or surrounding areas, this is despite 97 percent of our nation's land being considered rural. We no longer have to tap into our intrinsic knowledge of what is medicine or poison, or exercise our resourcefulness in seasonal hunting and gathering in order to get the food we need to stay alive. We also decrease our access to the natural resources, like clean air, and land for growing our own food.

Thankfully, our body has its own processing centers and janitorial service, and we don't have to consciously control our heartbeat, respiration, or other vital functions. The only owner's manual we'll ever need came built-in as our internal or circadian clock. It's impossible to turn off this clock or hit snooze, but we should still be aware of how it works in the background all the time, triggering the ideal times for eating, sleeping, physical movement, and creative and logical thinking.

Ancient and modern medicine have different concepts and terminology to describe this clock: Early science describes light-dark cycles, and today we talk about the twenty-four-hour clock. But all agree that going against the timing of nature can negatively impact our health.

The Ayurvedic Clock

The Ayurvedic clock gives doshic assignment to different times of day. As we saw in chapter 1, every dosha is responsible for different physiological functions, and this clock helps to reflect how different organs and systems have their peaks. Certain periods of day also take on different qualities, so if we know the dosha that corresponds to a specific time of day, we can be on the lookout for potential imbalances while also maximizing our ability to complete both conscious tasks and those that our body automatically performs.

The Ayurvedic clock is divided into six four-hour periods. Notice that the Ayurvedic approach to the time of day is exactly how we address the balance of our own dosha. To some degree, we want to play into its strengths, but we also need to be tuned into when we are doing too much.

6 AM–10 AM

Morning is kapha time: time to embrace strong earth qualities by participating in physical movement, manual labor, or personal hygiene. Because you're very grounded at this time of day, it also offers a good opportunity to work on projects that require endurance of mind. Journaling, dense or challenging reading, deep-cleaning your home, or going for a long bike ride or run are a few examples of ways you can play into the doshic qualities of the morning. On the flip side, the later you sleep into this time frame or the more inactive you are, the groggier you'll feel. Maybe you've been tempted to stay in bed when you naturally wake up at your normal time on a weekend, but because you don't have to be anywhere, you decide to sleep in. But then, when you finally decide to get up, you feel tired. You might think you had "too much sleep," but rather than excess sleep it's because of excess kapha—an accumulation of heavy energy—that's acting in opposition to the timekeeping of our internal clock.

10 AM–2 PM

Pitta presides over the middle of the day. It shouldn't be a surprise that the fire element is so closely associated with the peak of the sun. Like the sun, our digestion also burns hottest at this time, making it the best time to eat your biggest meal. And as pitta rules our analytical mind, we are best at tasks that require clear focus during these hours, such as doing your bookkeeping, organizing your calendar, or studying for an upcoming exam. But keep in mind, you don't want to combine too many pitta activities together. Choosing to eat while you work to get through the report your boss is waiting for will leave you feeling more agitated than balanced, and being hyperfocused on one thing without taking a break can result in burnout.

2 PM–6 PM

Vata reigns over the late afternoon and into early evening. Vata governs the nervous system, meaning you may feel a spike in your fight-or-flight response. This can lead to you having a creative peak during this time frame. Use it to your advantage by planning activities that involve free-form innovation and brainstorming. The orderly and analytical tasks you excelled at earlier in the day won't come as easily in the afternoon; however, you could have your best ideas for clever marketing campaigns, creative layouts for your current art projects, or a new design concept for your kitchen remodel. A word of caution: Similar to the agitation that can come from overloading pitta in the afternoon, abusing vata energy will leave you feeling tired and depleted with an inability to concentrate. It may seem contrary, but when you feel a draw to reenergize at this time of day with coffee or a hit of a sugary snack, do the opposite: take a walk outside, meditate, or take a ten-minute break.

6 PM–10 PM

We cycle back around to kapha for the evening (notice the hours are the same as morning, just PM). Since kapha represents strength and endurance, this could be your second choice for scheduling exercise and hygienic tasks that round out your day. Stay on the earlier side of the window, though, since this is also time we should be winding down for sleep. As a part of this preparation for rest, our digestion also slows. Thus, make dinner early and light, and try to avoid any stimulating activities after 8 PM, especially if it involves electronic devices that emit blue light, which tricks our mind into thinking it is still daytime.

10 PM–2 AM

A parallel to the middle of the day, the middle of the night is also governed by pitta. The fire at this later time is devoted to detoxification, liver function, revitalizing our skin, blood cleansing, and mental restoration. There could be the temptation to dive into work that requires more focus late at night (our pitta friends often have a predisposition to being night owls), but this would be misuse of the pitta energy. Ayurveda subscribes not only to the idea of getting a certain amount of sleep, but also to the idea of everyone sleeping during certain hours. This goes back to the connection between organ systems and the doshas: Remember pitta organs govern transformation, so allowing them to be restored during their night shift means we can use them more effectively during the day. And as much as we don't want to admit it, we aren't good multitaskers by nature. Choosing to stay awake too far past 10

PM could mean that you're diverting energy away from important body functions, making you less productive when nature says it's time it sink into your flow in the daylight.

2 AM–6 AM

The early morning takes on the doshic qualities of vata. This light and mobile period is when both your dreams and mind are most active. Though you are likely to be asleep for a good portion of this time, it is considered to be a most auspicious hour and the best time for spiritual practices, such as prayer or meditation. Buddhist monks, and members of other religious communities wake around 4 AM for this very reason. Ayurveda does recommend rising with the sun, not to be rigid or punishing; rather, it is a way to be more in sync with the day to come. If you are sleeping when the vata dosha and your internal clock are signaling your physiology to get moving—and I mean this quite literally, as we should always urinate first thing in the morning and this is the most natural time of day for bowel movements—the opportunity may pass you by. Unfortunately, there is no make up period for these things! But stay on the bright side, there are ways to adopt earlier wake times, even if you don't describe yourself as a natural morning person.

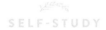

SELF-STUDY

Not only is timing important, but consistency is key. What time of day do you eat, sleep, and exercise? Are you consistent with your own schedule and with the Ayurvedic clock?

The Circadian Clock

With today's more advanced means and methods for research, modern medicine is now "proving" the connection between our internal cycles and the sun that Ayurvedic physicians, or *vaidyas*, have always known to be true. There's abundant evidence that light-dark cycles greatly affect human physiology.

Chronobiology, or circadian medicine, is a branch of Western medicine that studies our body's natural rhythms and how they repeat themselves in cycles. Most commonly known are circadian rhythms. The word *circadian* is derived from Latin words *circa*, meaning "about," and *dies*, meaning "day." A circadian rhythm or cycle describes our twenty-four-hour internal clock by which our physical, mental, and behavioral patterns are mapped. Other cycles last more than twenty-four hours, such as seasonal cycles, moon cycles, and the female menstrual cycle. These are called infradian rhythms. Cycles lasting shorter than a twenty-four-hour period are called ultradian rhythms; these are things like breathing cycles, our heartbeat, and the way we fluctuate in and out of REM and non-REM sleep.

Circadian cycles are primarily influenced by daylight; however, what and when we eat, our sleeping habits, and conducting our day in consistent or sporadic ways all impact our daily cycles. Eating at random times from one day to the next, or having erratic sleep times and amounts, are all causes for misalignment. Jet lag is a perfect example of how an abrupt versus gradual change in your schedule and circadian cycle can make you feel unwell. A version of this also happens on weekends when you stay out past your regular bedtime, aka "social jet lag." Our body rhythms are set to a predetermined internal clock, and when we deviate away from it, our bodies make their unhappiness known.

Circadian medicine is very much aligned with the Ayurvedic clock. While Ayurveda uses doshas and elements to explain our biological shifts throughout the day, circadian medicine speaks to the changes in organs and hormones over a twenty-four-hour cycle.

6 AM–12 PM

A natural release of cortisol, the infamous stress hormone, occurs around 6 AM and blood pressure slowly starts to increase. This is also the time of day when testosterone is the highest, and as a result, you'll peak in strength, energy, and alertness in the middle of this time frame. Though many people typically reach for stimulants to get themselves going early in the day, if you have your coffee too early, such as before 8 AM, it can add to the effects of your already naturally released cortisol. This is unfavorable, as it sends a signal to our body that we are under extreme stress and that it's time to go into survival mode. If you rely on caffeine, have it a little later, or try reducing the amount you consume by at least half.

12 PM–6 PM

We have the fastest reaction time and the best hand-eye coordination in the afternoon. Two main factors contribute to this: Afternoon is when lung function is optimal and when body temperature increases to its highest point in the twenty-four-hour cycle. While this may have made the afternoon a good time for our evolutionary ancestors to chase prey and evade predators, today it could make us better drivers or more competitive tennis partners. In part a result of our standard adult workday that requires us to keep pushing through tiredness, we might need stress relief at this time of day. It could be most advantageous to use our highly functioning respiratory system for mindful breathing practices.

6 PM–12 AM

Melatonin, one of the hormones that regulate our sleep cycle, is released between the hours of 9 PM and 10 PM. This signals to our body that it is time to sleep, in part so that our clock can run smoothly for another day. Blue light from electronics artificially suppresses melatonin because our body perceives it to be natural daylight. While taking melatonin supplements may help remedy insomnia by resetting your circadian clock, the best solution is to have lots of exposure to natural daylight throughout the day, and to limit the use of devices at night, especially after 6 PM.

12 AM–6 AM

As we sleep, our body naturally repairs and restores. We have our own self-regulating cleansing system that rids our body of waste and toxic substances; our liver is the primary organ that neutralizes harmful substances like alcohol, medications, or chemicals found in food. This natural detoxification process takes place during the night—but only if you are asleep. Our liver function begins to change from producing bile during the day to metabolizing toxins around 10 PM and continues its purifying work through 3 AM. This is our brain's time to be swept clean, too, as the flow of cerebrospinal fluid increases and moves any buildup of harmful waste from our brain cells. This helps you properly form memories and to allow you to think clearly the next day.

The Ayurvedic clock and the circadian clock may not exactly overlap, but they complement and support one another. If you were to design your day according to either clock, you'd find yourself waking and going to bed early, exercising toward the beginning or ending of the day, and having a hearty meal somewhere in between. Both emphasize the same underlying message: Our body is set to natural cycles, and disregard to these cycles consequentially results in illness.

Table 2. The Twenty-Four-Hour Ayurvedic and Circadian Clocks

TIME FRAME	AYURVEDIC DOSHA	AYURVEDA: PHYSIOLOGICAL FUNCTIONS	CIRCADIAN MEDICINE: PHYSIOLOGICAL FUNCTIONS	
6–10 AM	Kapha (water + earth)	Physical strength is greatest, absorption and assimilation, immunity is being built	Testosterone is at its peak in both men and women, strongest time of day, time when most efficiently burn fat, cortisol is released and increased	
10 AM–2 PM	Pitta (fire + water)	Digestive fire is at its peak, mental skills are sharpest	Mental alertness, blood pressure increases	
2–6 PM	Vata (ether + air)	Nervous system becomes more active, capacity for creativity increases	Reaction times are fastest, hand-eye coordination is at its best, lung function is at its best, blood pressure peaks	
6–10 PM	Kapha (water + earth)	Heaviness signals body and mind to settle down	Melatonin secretion, blood pressure begins to decrease, body temperature is highest	
10 PM–2 AM	Pitta (fire + water)	Detoxification process, liver function is high, metabolism is being controlled, adrenals and thyroid are being restored	Detoxification, skin cell turnover, organ restoration and repair	
2–6 AM	Vata (ether + air)	Nervous system starts to become active, vivid dreams occur, internal movement and elimination of waste	Brain restoration, memories form, deepest sleep, body temperature is lowest	

ACTIVITIES THAT ALIGN BEST WITH THIS TIME	COMMON MISUSE OF THIS TIME	COMMON PHYSICAL AND MENTAL IMBALANCES SEEN AT THIS TIME
Exercise, manual labor, activities that require mental or physical endurance	Sleeping too late, eating too heavy of a meal, not engaging in physical activity or exposure to daylight	Sluggishness, lethargy, feeling low
Eating your biggest meal, activities that require mental focus or acuity such as planning and organizing	Skipping lunch, working through lunch, vigorous exercise, engaging in activities that aren't healthy for the physical or emotional heart	Anger, frustration, excessive heat, mental burnout, indigestion
Leisure, immersion in nature, creative activities, meditation	Stimulants to boost energy, forcing activities that require focus, pushing through when tired	Low energy, inability to focus, hyperactivity
Winding down, family time, reading, gentle physical practices, self-care/ hygienic routines	Engaging with blue light from electronics, forcing self to stay awake, eating a too-large meal or biggest meal, eating past 8 PM.	Fatigue, difficulty staying awake, heavy feelings
Sleep	Starting new projects, using devices that emit blue light	Difficulty falling asleep, waking due to problem-solving mind, feeling hot
Sleep, wake before or with the sun, meditation, evacuation of bowels and bladder, hygienic self-care rituals	Stimulants like coffee consumed on an empty stomach	Waking due to anxiety or fleeting thoughts, feeling cold, or the need to urinate

PART 2

Rituals for Everyone to Embrace

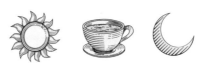

CHAPTER 4

Your Day Defines You

How Rituals Play a Role in Your Well-Being

You go away on vacation, where you've unplugged and blissed out, only to come back and regret that your time away has gotten you out of your groove—the place where you thrive at home, at work, and in health. You tell your friends and colleagues that you'll be back on top of things when you're back into your routine. Once you find your groove, you feel lighter, clearer, and more self-aware. No wonder Stella was looking to get hers back.

Though this familiar storyline may have you nodding in agreement, you may not have taken the time to truly acknowledge how the structure of your day impacts your health and the life you're manifesting. When your "fulfilling" life of career, family, and fun is feeling over-filled; convenience and multitasking replace your daily anchors and regard for mindful transitions; and your mind often moves onto the next task before the current one is completed. Looking for the fastest route to feeling good again, you turn to "superfoods" with the highest nutritional content, or to the latest trending workout that promises to make you lose weight fast or give your muscles the most tone, only to be left with practices that are fleeting or not sustainable.

These initiatives can certainly provide a quick fix. I've leaned on them myself, and countless people who come in and out of my office have, too. But quick fixes, no mater how well-intentioned, aren't viable for long-term health. This is a bit of good news, since it means that it's not your fault if a supplement or other wellness trend isn't working. The technology that was designed to make life easier has also managed to make working, eating, exercising, and sleeping at any hour easier. This goes against when our body would naturally be signaled to do these things, and instead of feeling better, we feel worse. We can obtain food at all times of year and from all over the world, and we can even manufacture food—injecting it with "healthy" additives so much that it's no longer technically food. Similarly, the very devices that were meant to keep us connected have disconnected us from the energy we were once closest to: nature. The result is a world you experience more often by staring at a tiny screen than through physical immersion.

The way out of this cycle is easier than you think. Rather than relying on external, man-made cues, we can sync with our deeper instinctual clock, to know and feel the best opening, closing, and general design for our days. Adding more awareness to the way you conduct your day not only gives you an outline for health, but also allows you to connect with your intuition so you supply yourself with what you need in each moment, not just what your phone's calendar or an online post says it's time to do.

And when your daily anchors are consistent, cyclical, and meaningful, they take on a ritualistic feel. Acting as a container for your life, scheduled self-care builds a sturdy foundation for health, and you don't have to be tricked into eating your peas for it to happen. With intentional routine, you're in the prime position for achieving your goals with unwavering energy and focus. Furthermore, if you're able to synchronize your watch with nature's, you'll optimize the functions of your physiology and increase the potency of your actions.

Ayurveda's overall mission is to create this synchronicity so we live in harmony with nature and the cycles that exist within it. It defines health as having a balanced constitution, healthy tissues, properly functioning digestion and excretion of waste, and a state of well-being in our senses, our mind, and our soul. The rituals you'll learn about in chapters 5 through 7 are the processes recommended for achieving exactly that. In part, they ensure self-care is part of our everyday activities. But beyond the rituals' content, their structure and consistency is just as, if not more, important for achieving balance. Our current lack of attention to cycles, routine, and nature has left our society as a whole with a vata imbalance. If you or your peers, coworkers, friends, and family experience conditions such as anxiety, insomnia, and indigestion, this may apply to you. That makes the need to return to cyclical, grounding practices even more urgent today.

Rituals have long been used in other cultures around the world as rites of passage, and as events that pass on knowledge from our ancestors for health and survival. Rituals have been the temporal, spiritual, and healthful landmarks that make things feel special and give our life meaning. Even in modern times, many such markers are embedded in our childhood memories. If you recall the happenings from when you were growing up, you'll likely note how clearly demarcated the passage of time was, from the hours of our school days to milestone birthdays. Meeting a friend at her locker before class, a family pizza or game night every Friday, studying for finals, the changes in holiday decorations in your house or town . . . they all had their own distinct vibe, separate even from positive or negative associations. Whatever your personal rituals were, their presence contributed to the way you embodied the passage of time or a season. They created a sense of anticipation or closure, helped you establish a place in nature, and helped you to prepare for what was to come.

Consider what rituals exist for you today. Unfortunately, as the world becomes more digitized, we see disrupted cycles and fewer constants. We meet people in person less often, we struggle to recognize cues from

> **SELF-STUDY**
>
> What current routines, rituals, and traditions do you honor? Do you have a morning, midday, and evening routine? Imagine your ideal day— what daily rituals could align with this ideal day?

the sun and seasons, and our intuition and senses have atrophied when it comes to making decisions regarding our health. There may be a general upkeep of some traditions, as our holidays and weather are still roughly the same, but society's praise for busyness lends to dishonor for slowing down and having space.

How Your Dosha Plays a Role in Rituals and Routine

One of the most advantageous things about knowing your dosha or your constitution is that you can predict things that would have required years of self-study to otherwise determine. Your vulnerabilities become as clear as day. Having this knowledge is not a guarantee that you can prevent any illness, live completely stress-free, or avoid all potential setbacks, but you can be better prepared when such things occur. Think of it like packing for a vacation. You can check the weather and take everything you think you might need, but there could still be a rain shower when all you were expecting was sun. Your dosha would be the thing telling you you might want to bring an umbrella, just in case.

If you know your needs and tendencies, you'll be better informed for the future. Mirroring the three Ayurvedic constitutions, there are three general mentalities that affect how you approach rituals, routine, and structure. You may find yourself a solid fit for one classification, or you may notice that there is some overlap for you, as is the case with the doshas themselves.

Vata: You need structure, but you resist structure.

The vata dosha, the constitution of ether and air, is in constant movement. If by nature you crave change and spontaneity, it's also likely you will naturally avoid routine. But like gases, if there is not a container to define the vata dosha, it can't take on a shape or form. That means vatas can benefit from structure the most.

If you struggle with making decisions, have trouble focusing on a single task, or find it difficult to make commitments, this may be an indicator of your internal inclination to resist structure, or your current need for implementing routine. When you notice yourself contracting around the idea of bringing consistency and set actions into your day, remember this: Structure creates room for play, and having a schedule or routine means there are fewer times when you will have to make the decisions you naturally resist. When you are rooted and pay respect to the beginning and end cycles of a day, you'll be more effective and efficient in between. Thus, there will ultimately be more room to embrace what you need in the moment.

Pitta: You love systems and routine, but you risk being overly structured.

The pitta dosha, the constitution of fire and water, thrives on organization, preparedness, following directions, and adhering to rituals. As a lovers of logic, they have their systems in place. Pittas know what they want and they like to be in control. They believe that their way is the best—and want everyone to agree.

There's reason to applaud your great discipline and willpower, but there will be consequences—if not now, then eventually—when routines rule you, instead of your ruling the routines. When you only live inside your container, with your planner or schedule like blinders, there's a possibility that you lean toward being too rigid, lack enough free time in your day to restore, or even turn moments of self-care into more of an agenda than an act of agenda-free self-love. If there's allure in the idea of adding another challenge, checklist, or more things to your planner, be on the lookout for stringency.

Kapha: Your routine needs an occasional shake-up, but you are averse to change.

The water and earth elements that comprise the kapha dosha make it a difficult constitution to budge. Kaphas, whether it be from nostalgia or discomfort with uncertainty, can easily get stuck in their ways. Doing the same thing and unwavering no matter the circumstances, you don't want to put forth energy to make a change you don't feel is necessary. Yet this static dosha benefits from vigorous activities, and mixing things up brings balance.

While no change should be forced (and quite honestly, it can't be), keep in mind that things accumulate, and our requirements for fulfillment don't remain the same as we ourselves grow and change.

SELF-STUDY

Historically, how do you respond to routine or starting new ones? What would be helpful for you in maintaining daily rituals?

A bowl of ice cream before bed may have served you well as a kid, and midnight coffee runs may have felt great during your college years—but are your current needs the same as they were then? Probably not. Our internal and external environments change, and without the flexibility or willingness to change with them, we can become unwell.

We all experience our own personal struggles with maintaining routine and rituals. Though you can find inspiration through others, what is most important is looking within yourself for the approach that is best for you.

CHAPTER 5

Daily Rituals

Practices for an Intentional Start to Your Day,
and Easeful Transitions Throughout

One of Ayurveda's strongest roles is to prevent disease and maintain health, whereas modern medicine's strength is to induce healing after illness has already occurred. Each approach is necessary in a comprehensive health model; we need both preventive and emergency health care. Ayurveda and modern medicine agree that health is more than merely the absence of disease, but the act of achieving a balance of sound mind, body, and spirit. Not only is what we do to achieve this important, but also the timing of our actions is crucial.

Prevention comes very naturally to Ayurveda. Embedded in its tradition is an extensive daily routine, with the implication that someone who practices a routine will live in good health. The word used to describe such conduct is *swasthavritta*. This term represents something more complex than dubbing a routine "healthy," since it stands for how we abide by our own nature and the duties required to establish such a state.

The Ayurvedic routine is multifaceted and includes recommendations for daily (6 AM to 6 PM), nightly (6 PM to 10 PM), and seasonal routines. Respectively, these are referred to as *dinacharya*, *ratricharya*, and *ritucharya*. In ancient Ayurvedic texts, you'll find these rituals detailed beautifully beyond a checklist. Worth more than the sum of their parts, these ritual sets are effective because of their combined timing, sequence, and intention.

Now that you've identified some of your current patterns in chapter 2 and tendencies toward routine in chapter 4, you can find out how your day compares to how Ayurveda recommends aligning our days. We'll start with dinacharya, or Ayurveda's daily routine, which is safe for everyone to adopt—though occasional contraindications and modifications may be needed to suit one's constitution or imbalance. Dinacharya is the lengthiest set of rituals because it involves steps to refresh ourselves after nightly detoxification during sleep, and for ensuring that we can begin our day with sound mind and body. In our modern world, some of the components are easier to integrate than others. It's impossible to speak for those who wrote the texts thousands of years ago, but it seems they held more regard for reserving time for self-care than for working. With the many demands on our time to produce more, and more quickly, there may not actually be enough hours to do it all. Don't let that prevent you from trying anything, though: The emphasis will always be on doing what you can and when, versus worrying about what you can't do and inconsistencies.

The standard dinacharya involves these rituals:

Ancient Ayurvedic texts advise that you rise before the sun, one and a half hours prior to be exact. This is because it is considered to be the most auspicious time of day, making it the best time for meditation, taking in knowledge, or self-study. With all due respect to these ancient authors, this first suggested ritual of the day can often seem too traditional (especially for night owls), and maybe not the most realistic one to tackle first. Unless you have a solid reason, such as getting to a job or taking someone to the airport, you most likely don't see this time of day and aren't about to start. Understood. Still, it is worth considering what you could gain from these early (or earlier) morning hours.

Embracing the vata period of the morning puts you on track to get things moving. It is the most natural time of day to eliminate from both bowels and bladder, according to Ayurveda and Western medicine. Getting out of bed early could mean less variability in the efficiency and ease of your digestion.

Waking with the sun also provides you with seasonal flexibility. In the summer, the earlier sunrise and extended day can make you feel liberated. You wake earlier so that you have more time to work, play, or whatever activities the summer season has you craving. In the winter, you're afforded more rest with the later sunrise, and the shorter days that allow for more overall time for sleep.

MEDITATE

Whether you call it prayer, meditation, or mental hygiene, mindful stillness comes to us most easily in the early morning. Aside from morning being an auspicious time of day (think: happy thoughts), at this time our mind hasn't had a lot of time to start racing so meditating with fewer mental fluctuations isn't as challenging. Many of us envision meditation as sitting completely motionless on a cushion in a quiet room with your legs in a pretzel. You don't have to be in that idealized posture; instead, let your practice meet you where you are. If simply sitting up in bed with your eyes closed for a few minutes works for you, go for it. If you feel like you need a tutorial and have an app or a guided meditation to listen to, use it. The practice, not the outcome or the method, is what matters.

CLEAN YOUR TONGUE

Before eating, drinking, brushing your teeth, or swishing with oil or mouthwash (see page 67), scrape your tongue. This isn't only about oral hygiene; similar to our skin, the tongue is a big indicator of your digestive health and more.

The first step is to examine your tongue before anything could interfere with what's on it from the night. The main thing to look out for is the coating. It can tell you whether you have inefficient *agni*, or digestive fire, which results in *ama*. This is a toxic buildup of what you are not digesting, in both the body and the mind. Sometimes you can see it, or even smell it, in the case of your tongue. Other times it isn't visible, as when emotional experiences you haven't processed build up.

You may not always find a notable layer of coating on your tongue or scrape much off of it, but if you're dealing with some digestive woes, there is a pretty good chance your tongue will tell you something. These properties will give you the inside scoop on what's happening further down the tract.

Location

If there is a layer across the back of your tongue only, this indicates that you aren't fully eliminating with each bowel movement and that waste is hiding out in your colon. Coating that is primarily at the middle of the tongue is a sign that there are toxins or unabsorbed or undigested food accumulating in your stomach and small intestine.

Color

If the coating is frothy or a light brown color, this is indicative of a vata imbalance (accumulated air element) and a low or variable digestive fire. Reducing raw or drying food (crackers, chips, beans, or coffee) will be balancing. A yellow, orange, or green coating means that pitta (fire) is elevated and your digestive fire is burning too hot. Spicy, sour, and salty foods should be reduced. Lastly, a whitish coating shows that kapha (earth) has increased, showing evidence of a sluggish digestion and a need to lay low on food that can be heavy, like dairy and sweets.

Thickness

If you continually (every day over the course of two weeks) find a thick coating, you are accumulating ama. It's important to be aware of ama, as the material will cause blockage, stagnation, and a weakened immunity. Your tongue is one of the first places you can spot ama, no matter if it is from emotional or dietary origin.

After assessing what is happening in your body by examining your tongue, you start cleaning. Instead of using your toothbrush, invest in a tongue cleaner. It's worth the splurge (of around $10 or less). What a tongue cleaner can do that a toothbrush can't is make a full sweep of your tongue and show you exactly what you're scraping off. They also come in a variety of metals that complement your dosha: Silver is a cooling metal and also used to improve strength, so it's best for vata and pitta, whereas copper is the metal of choice for kapha because it is said to be tonifying (meaning it can replenish and bring energy to tissues or organs). Stainless steel is a good choice for all doshas. These metals also have antibacterial properties, so even though you do need to clean the scraper, it inherently resists the germs that bristles would easily harbor.

Start at the back of your tongue, and use gentle pressure as you scrape down the center, clearing off the layer of toxins that accumulated during the night. Repeat on the left and right sides of the tongue, always moving, from back to front. Repeat this center, side, side method a few times, letting what you are scraping off accumulate before rinsing the tongue scraper clean. Note that cleaning your tongue is separate from oil pulling/swishing (see page 67), which should occur after eating breakfast.

When the coating is removed from your tongue, you're immediately given a better ability to perceive tastes. This is essential for healthy digestion because everything we consume breaks down differently. Having an adequate sense of taste is like announcing to your body, "Incoming, sweet!" or "Watch out for the salt bomb!," which lets it better prepare to process what you're eating. Not to mention, the practice of tongue cleaning gets you into the routine of simply looking at your tongue to understand more about your current digestive health, so you can stay on top of symptoms that might not yet have arisen elsewhere in the body.

RINSE YOUR FACE AND EYES

A splash of water or spritz with a plant hydrosol (water with plant essences, such as rose or cucumber can be the perfect wake-up call. If you struggle with feeling sluggish or having a puffy face in the morning, move this part of your routine closer to the time you wake. You'll feel more alert and ready to carry out the rest of your rituals.

To be even more attentive, add in the basic practice of rinsing your eyes. Unless you wear corrective lenses or have dealt with a specific eye condition, you likely don't spend a lot of time caring for your eyes. And in some cases, that may only stretch as far as (hopefully) washing or changing your contact lenses. With our excessive use of screens and exposure to environmental toxins, this is an area we can all improve.

As you would take caution with what you are eating or putting on your skin, you must be extra careful with what you are using to wash your eyes. While the bare bones approach of running water over your eyes in the shower or when rinsing your face could work in a pinch, using an eyewash cup and dedicated solutions can give you more comfort and increased results. If you are using water, filtered water works best. Other solutions that have an affinity for healing the eyes must also be as pure as possible. For example, the herbal formula *triphala* (see Glossary of Herbs, page 267) can be made into a decoction or tea and used as an eyewash. When doing so, not only should you look for pure, organic triphala, but also you'll need to be sure it has been sufficiently strained and there aren't any remaining particulates that could scratch your eye. Rose hydrosol is also excellent for hydrating and soothing eyes, but again, look for the best quality you can find.

RINSE YOUR NASAL PASSAGES WITH A NETI POT

If you suffer from allergies or recurring upper-respiratory infections, or are simply enamored with the idea of taking clear, full deep breaths, add a neti pot to your shopping list.

Nasal rinsing, or *jala neti*, is a practice that cleanses, soothes, and frees the nasal passages of obstruction, improving overall respiratory health. A neti pot is a vessel that looks a lot like a teapot and allows for gentle nasal irrigation. A saltwater solution is used for the rinse; it is poured into one nostril and exits out the other. Though you can find alternatives for nasal rinses, they are often in squeeze bottles. But as with a tongue cleaner, a true neti pot is worth the investment, as it won't be as forceful as the squeeze bottle and reduces use of disposable plastics. Neti pots are mainstream enough to be available in the personal care sections of most natural grocery stores and pharmacies.

To start, mix about ¼ teaspoon of non-iodized salt with about eight ounces (240 ml) warm distilled or filtered water. You can buy salt specifically for a neti pot: This variety dissolves easily, won't cause any burning sensations, and won't have any preservatives that you already try to avoid in your food. Make sure the water and vessel are sterile so that you aren't directly introducing any bacteria or viruses into your sinuses.

Either over the sink or when in the shower, place the spout of your neti pot into one nostril. Tilt your head forward slightly and begin to tip both the pot and your head toward the side of the free nostril. Do this until you feel the saline solution flowing into one nostril and out the other. Breathe through your mouth. Bring your head back to the neutral position and remove the spout. Breathe out through your nose several times to be sure the solution has fully cleared. Repeat this entire process on the other side.

No matter how happy the woman on the box looks performing it, using a neti pot can be a little uncomfortable until you have gotten used to it. If you're having difficulty getting the water to flow through one side, making you feel like your condition is getting worse (or giving you bad memories of diving into a swimming pool), give it a rest. Note that neti, or any other type of sinus rinse, doesn't couple so well with the practice of administering oil to your nasal passages, called *nasya* (coming up on page 69). As you know, oil and water don't mix; unless you're certain no water is left behind, oil and water can be left to mingle in your sinuses, ultimately acting as an aid in harboring allergens or illnesses.

DRINK WARM WATER

After a night of restoration and detoxification, your body could use a little assistance in getting ready to receive fuel for the day.

The first thing that you should consume, before coffee or any kind of solid food, is water.

Ayurveda would dissuade you from drinking copious amounts of water, or any other liquid, at once because it will extinguish your digestive fire. However, drinking more water at one sitting first thing in the morning can do the opposite. Water, particularly warm to hot water, primes your digestive system; remember the rule about liquid temperatures from chapter 2. Consuming a full sixteen ounces (480 ml) after you wake up will promote the proper elimination and breakdown of what you're going to eat during the day. At all other times of day, sharpen your sipping skills.

There are ways to amplify your water's cleansing properties, such as drinking from a copper mug. Before you go to bed, fill a copper cup (make sure it is copper on the inside, too) with water. The water will become infused with a therapeutic amount of copper during the night, so when you consume it in the morning, you're drinking something more medicinal than plain water. Larger amounts of copper can be toxic, but in this practice, it acts as a blood purifier, helps to reduce inflammation, alleviates joint pain, and aids in clarifying skin.

Lemon can also elevate your morning water-drinking game. Though lemon itself is acidic, it is alkalizing once inside the body, so adding a slice of lemon or a squeeze of fresh lemon juice to your water increases your body's pH to an environment better equipped to fight disease (we are naturally in a slightly alkaline state, around 7.4 on the pH scale). Lemon can also be a digestive aid, as it helps break down fat and can increase the flow of bile.

It's best to allow some buffer time between drinking a sizable amount of water and eating, so after drinking, make sure you wait at least fifteen minutes before breakfast.

If you have your finger on the pulse of the wellness scene, the practice of oil pulling, or *gandusha*, isn't new to you. This modern trend actually originated with Ayurveda.

Oil pulling is called such because oil has an ability to pull away impurities; it's a favorite tool in Ayurveda, as we'll see. When used orally, it helps to clean and whiten your teeth, but it also has deeper therapeutic effects. The practice is said to strengthen facial muscles, provide maximum taste and relish in food, firmly root and straighten teeth, and prevent dryness of the lips, mouth, and throat.

There are two ways to approach oil pulling within Ayurvedic tradition, both are done after you clean your tongue. One is to swish a little bit (about 1 tablespoon) oil in your mouth for a few minutes, as if using mouthwash, and the other is to fill your mouth with oil and to hold it still for up to twenty minutes. Swishing is more practical for an everyday routine, but holding the oil can be a more grounding practice and is suitable to those who have vata imbalances or conditions aggravated by excessive physical or mental movement. In either scenario, spit the oil out into a trash can when you are done to avoid clogging pipes and drains.

The best oil for this depends on the mouth it's cleaning. In general, when you see the word *oil* in Ayurveda, you can mentally replace it with "sesame oil." Sesame is the king of oils because it is the only one that can reach and nourish all tissues. It is too heating for consumption in the summer, or for those who have a lot of fire in their constitution or have fiery imbalances, but because you aren't consuming the oil when pulling, it typically is OK for everyone to use in this way. Be sure to use pure sesame oil, not toasted, and always prefer organic and unrefined oil for this use.

If choosing not to use sesame oil, you can look for preformulated oils with herbs that have been created specifically for swishing. You could also try plain sunflower or grapeseed oil from the grocery store for something neutral, or you can use coconut oil for an over-all cooling effect, especially in the summer.

BRUSH YOUR TEETH

What with tongue cleaning and oil swishing, you may be won-dering where brushing your teeth—what most of us know as the primary form of oral hygiene—fits into the mix. In Ayurveda, it is preferred after both of these steps. First, you examine your tongue to see how well your digestion is working, and then oil pulling second, which helps to soften any impurities in your mouth and remove plaque from between your teeth to aid the work of your toothbrush and floss.

Though there isn't any specific warning against using a typical commercial toothpaste, Ayurveda traditionally promotes using a tooth powder. A combination of herbs known to be beneficial for oral hygiene, such as neem, triphala, fennel, and licorice, are often used. The powder can be used on your toothbrush as you would toothpaste, or it can also be used by scrubbing your teeth and gums with your finger; you just won't generate the foam you do with commercial brands. Rinse with warm water, and get ready to greet the day with a clean smile.

OIL YOUR NASAL CAVITIES AND SINUSES

The nasal passages are a direct pathway to the brain, and the practice of *nasya*, or the administration of oil to the nose and sinuses, helps to nourish that important trajectory.

Nasya might be right for you if you experience dry sinuses, recurring sinus infections, allergies, or difficulty in settling your mind. As the oil helps to lubricate your sinuses, it keeps them from becoming raw and inflamed, an environment that can be a breeding ground for infections. Oil is also nourishing to our nervous system, which helps explain why holding oil in the mouth can be good for vata.

This is because the substance that covers each nerve, called the myelin sheath, is made of fats, but also because oil is balancing to vata and the ether and air elements that govern the nervous system.

If you're using an oil that was formulated with nasya in mind, it will have herbs such as brahmi, bacopa, skullcap, or gotu kola (see Glossary of Herbs, page 267), which help to nourish the nervous system, aid in improving memory and concentration, and reduce congestion. These are all things that oil alone can help with, but the herbs help to give it an extra boost. If you'd like to try it with a basic oil before buying something extra that you may not be fully committed to, use organic sesame oil.

To perform nasya, use a bottle with a dropper. Lie back and drop anywhere from three to five drops into one nostril. Close the opposite nostril and take a deep breath. Repeat this process on the other side. Stay reclined for a few minutes, or until you feel that the oil has moved into your sinuses and isn't hanging out in your nasal passageway.

This practice can take some getting used to. It won't leave you with the water-up-the-nose feeling that nasal rinses like a neti pot's can; however, it can create some drainage in your throat. If you experience this, spit it out. Additionally, if you don't tip your head back the appropriate amount, you might notice that the oil doesn't make it too far, leaving you with some oil leakage each time you drop your head forward.

You may find it beneficial to reserve your nasya ritual for later in the day, as it can make you more focused and alert. If you have a time of day other than the morning that you practice breathing exercises, implementing nasya prior to breathwork can help the oil move deeper into the nasal passageway and sinus cavities. Choosing to do this at night is OK, too, but make sure you allow yourself enough awake time post-nasya that you don't fall asleep with oil drainage at the back of your throat.

DRY-BRUSH YOUR BODY

Ayurvedic dry-brushing is called *garshana*. Typically done with raw silk gloves, it can also be performed using a body brush with natural bristles. The practice is always done before showering or applying any type of oil, cream, or lotion.

On a superficial level, this practice sloughs away any dry skin to prepare your body to hydrate through external oil massage. But on a deeper level, dry-brushing has a profound effect on the lymphatic system, an important part of our immunity that is only starting to get the attention that it deserves.

Briefly, the lymphatic system regulates the immune system and removes waste by transporting lymph and any blood that remains in the interstitial fluid. The direction of this movement is toward the heart. This is essentially our drainage system. It's important for our pipes and drains to stay open and fluid because they are helping to track waste through our body so that it can be removed.

Dry-brushing assists this process because it increases circulation. And when performed in coordination with the movement of the lymphatic system—toward the heart—it helps move lymph along its natural path. Once again, we are using rituals to enhance the body's ability to do what it is designed to do.

Thus, dry-brushing starts at your extremities. Use invigorating, long, methodical strokes as you move from your feet up your legs toward your torso, then from your hands up your arms toward your chest. Use circular strokes around joints and move the brush in a clockwise direction around your abdomen, back, and heart.

Dry-brushing is stimulating, and you may find that it reduces any sluggish or heavy feelings you experience. On the other hand, if you're feeling overstimulated, it's best to discontinue this practice or pick it up at another time.

PRACTICE SELF-MASSAGE WITH OIL

Dreamy, *magical*, and *soothing* are words that come to mind with the ritual of *abhyanga*, or oil massage. Among the many beneficial elements of the Ayurvedic self-care regimen, abhyanga stands out as having some of the most incredible, tangible effects.

Abhyanga is the practice of applying warm oil to your body through a gentle and methodical massage, prior to a bath or shower. If dry-brushing is part of your routine, the oil massage comes after that.

Start by heating ¼ to ½ cup (60 to 120 ml) of oil in a glass container, either by placing the container in hot water or running it underneath the faucet. You could also use a designated oil warmer, which heats the oil in a metal vessel using a candle. Warm oil will help to open your pores, allowing the oil to move into the tissue where it can be most nourishing.

Like with dry-brushing, you'll begin at your feet and hands and move toward your heart. Use circular motions around your joints and long strokes along arms and legs. Apply in a circular, clockwise motion across your abdomen, back, and chest. You can pay special attention to areas of concern, spending more time on your joints if they cause you pain or on your abdomen if you have upset digestion.

Theoretically, abhyanga will have the strongest effect if done in a warm, steamy room and when the oil is left on the skin for about twenty minutes. The reason is that Ayurvedic anatomy names seven layers of tissues, and it takes about twenty minutes to penetrate them all. If you are warm or can induce sweating while covered in oil, it is more likely that your pores will open and allow the medicine to move in. In today's world, that amount of time may seem like forever, so you can either choose to make this a weekly ritual, during which you can use abhyanga as a meditation and won't feel rushed, or shorten the ritual; even if you allow the oil to soak in for only five minutes, that isn't wasted time.

The oil used is chosen based on your constitution, the season, or the healing properties you need at a given time. Plain base oils or herb-infused oils are both fine. When you have a predominant amount of vata, or during the fall, you'll select warming and grounding sesame oil. If pitta or fire is abundant, and also during the summer, opt for something cooling, like coconut or sunflower oil. Kapha, or the earth and water elements that dominate in winter and spring, need something invigorating, and mustard seed oil is perfect for this.

As you might imagine, this practice takes care of dry skin in a jiffy—yet there are myriad other benefits as well. Ayurvedic texts say that those who use oil will ward off old age, be bestowed good vision, sleep well, and have strong, healthy skin. And since your skin is the largest organ of the body, it makes sense to use this as a means for administering medicine via herb-infused oil.

Self-massage has the ability to provide calm in times that are hectic, and security in moments of anxiety or vulnerability. In fact, even the translation of the word can make you feel hopeful. The Sanskrit word for oiling oneself is *snehana*, which also means "to love." Abhyanga is considered to be one of the greatest acts of self-love.

WHICH OIL DO I CHOOSE?

Oil is used extensively in Ayurveda, so it's best to find a resource for the oils that are appropriate for you. When you are reading about oil in recipes or directions for self-care and a specific oil isn't mentioned, it's safe to assume it is referring to one of the two most revered oils: sesame oil or ghee. There are reasons why you might choose another oil, such that sesame can be too heating for pitta dosha, so use this chart to guide you.

DOSHA	OIL
Vata	Sesame, ghee, sunflower, almond, avocado, walnut, castor, flaxseed, jojoba
Pitta	Coconut, ghee, sunflower, olive, avocado, jojoba
Kapha	Sesame, sunflower, ghee, mustard seed, safflower, almond, corn, flaxseed

As with many things in Ayurveda, exercise is meant to be personalized based on the season and your constitution, mood, and current state of health. The best time of day for all doshas to exercise is before 10 AM, or between 6 and 8 PM. And the duration? It depends how much you sweat. By Ayurvedic standards, one is to exercise to the point of perspiration on their forehead and armpits, assuming that there is also increased respiration. This idea may not jive with the high-intensity, hard-core gym-goers out there, but the rationale behind it is worth entertaining. It leaves us to assume that the primary aim of exercise at the time of Ayurveda's incarnation was to open sweat channels. It also allows us to question whether intensity is always better. Exercise is a type of controlled stress, but your nervous system can't differentiate if you are running for fitness or if you're sprinting away from a lion. The fight-or-flight response will be the same: increased heart rate, blood pressure, and breathing rate, and slowed digestion.

Exercising to complement your internal and external environment shouldn't seem like a radical concept. It's important to maintain cardiovascular endurance and muscular tone, but it could be argued that your overall state of health will also influence those things, not just going through the motions of fitness. If you are already under an extreme amount of stress, adding more high-intensity movement won't have the desired effects. Choosing more leisurely exercise, like restorative yoga or gentle walking, can keep you moving and sufficiently energized but without overtaxing your nervous system or promoting an imbalance of stress hormones in the long run. On the other hand, if you've had extended periods of being sedentary, unmotivated, or generally low-energy, or if the weather has you feeling sludgy or heavy (such as deep in winter or in the rainy spring), choose a workout with more vigor.

You'll notice, as these items of our daily routine are listed in sequential order, that exercise traditionally comes *after* oiling but before bathing. This is so the warmth and circulation created through movement can help our body more easily take in the nutrients of the oil. It's OK if this sequence doesn't work for you or just plain sounds like a soggy mess, but if you do decide to give it a try, wear old clothes that you don't mind getting oil-stained and remember that you'll be extra slippery!

BATHE

Your current morning shower may make you feel like you have a new lease on life, but Ayurveda has some guidelines surrounding this hygienic task you thought you mastered as a child.

The first regards timing. It's recommended that you don't bathe immediately after eating. One can only assume the old saying about not swimming after you've eaten stemmed from a similar theory: It has to do with digestion. In fact, it is best to not participate in anything that would increase your circulation, such as exercise or massage, at least one hour after eating. After you've consumed any amount of food, blood should be moving to the organs that aid in digestion. A hot shower or bath would counteract this by moving blood to your extremities. By Ayurvedic standards, a shower comes after both oiling and exercise and before you eat anything.

Another concept that may be new to many people is the limited use of soap. Even the best, most moisturizing soap tends to have a drying quality that strips away your skin's natural barrier. While you should still soap the places most likely to collect dirt or bacteria, like the underarms, feet, and genitals, try to avoid using it all over your skin. If this seems like a radical shift for you, have peace of mind in knowing that the oil will trap dirt particles that the water will then rinse away. For a compromise, try at least oiling your skin before you shower to get the process going, as suggested in the section about abhyanga (pages 72–74).

Consider as well the temperature of water. Cold showers are said to be revitalizing and can create a toning effect for our skin and muscles, whereas warmer showers increase blood flow and open our pores. So, which do you choose? First, if you have an imbalance, go with a temperature that will help to pacify: choose warm water for vata, cool to cold water for pitta, and the warmest for kapha. If you're not experiencing an imbalance or on the verge of one, let your shower temperature match what is needed with the season: choose cool for summer, warm for fall into winter, and the warmest for the spring, since warmer showers are more drying and we need the increased circulation this time of year. If you can't decide, lukewarm water is always a safe choice. Showers should be brief, five minutes or less, making it easier to adapt to a temperature that is cooler or warmer than your body's natural temperature.

Lastly, hot water, and heat in general, shouldn't be applied to your head. Used in this way, heat is said to be bad for our eyes, brain, and heart, and can drain us of energy. Try using lukewarm or cool water when washing your hair, wrapping a cool damp towel around your head if you are in a steam room or sauna, and letting your hair air-dry instead of using a hair dryer.

Although breakfast should always come after exercise and bathing in *dinacharya*, the earlier you eat, the better. (Are you starting to see why waking up early is useful?)

According to Ayurveda, we want to honor breakfast because of how it primes us for the actual most important meal of the day, lunch. Not to promote skipping a meal, but if you're not very hungry in the morning, listen to your gut and wait. For those who don't have strong hunger, baked or stewed fruit is a wonderful, simple option to tide you over until midday. If you look forward to your morning meal, opt for something heartier, like cooked oatmeal. Keep in mind the domino effect of delaying your breakfast too long, though: Your body needs about four to six hours to process food between meals; thus, delaying your breakfast equates to delaying your lunch, and then your dinner, and before you know it it's 11 PM and you're eating popcorn and nachos while watching Netflix, or sending out just one more email in the blue-light glow of your phone.

Everyone, no matter the season or their dosha, can take a pass on a frozen smoothie first thing in the morning. The intense cold puts out your digestive fire, which means frozen drinks actually aren't favorable at any time of day.

It's also not advisable for any dosha to have coffee on an empty stomach. The acidity is too much to mix straight with your stomach's natural acids, and if caffeinated, it's likely to be too much for your nervous system to handle and result in a major case of the jitters.

The food industry has done all it can to make breakfast easy for people to eat on the go. But I suggest you try sitting and not going anywhere while eating any meal. You have time, I promise. It typically takes no longer than ten to fifteen minutes to eat, and if it's taking you longer than twenty minutes, you're probably eating too much, talking too much, or doing something other than eating. For all the time you take to select the food

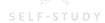

that is most nutritious for you, you owe it to yourself to relax and enjoy it. By slowly chewing and savoring each bite, and being grateful for the food itself along with those who helped it get to your plate, you can ensure all your meals are mindful.

Honoring the Midday Transition

There isn't a named set of Ayurvedic rituals for the middle of the day like there is for the morning, night, and seasons. Nevertheless, this juncture of AM and PM has great significance in achieving balance. During this time, when the sun peaks and many notice a change in their energy, mood, and ability to focus, a midday routine could prove to be life-changing.

Midday rituals all relate to the observation of transitions. Transitions offer you an opportunity to salute the end of one wave and welcome the beginning of another. They provide you with the tools you need to help you assess your previous steps and inform your future decisions. Transitions have also been proven to be a good time to develop new habits.

Midday routines can give our nervous system a reboot. While the nervous system is naturally self-regulating and shifts between sympathetic (fight or flight) to parasympathetic (rest and digest) modes on its own, a deliberate respite from busyness can usher in a needed reset. For most schoolchildren, midday or afternoon is typically the time for recess, snacks, or naps—essentially anything the teacher might need to do to wrangle and refocus the class. Adults need the same thing, but somewhere between primary school and the working world it was drilled into us that productivity is king, so we push through the day without respite. Our physiology is asking for a time-out, but we hold tight to our ability to mentally override nature. Although this nonstop mentality is now socially and corporately more acceptable than taking a grown-up recess, it also means our body stays in survival mode even when danger isn't afoot.

The most natural time for a pause during the day is lunch, which Ayurveda considers to be the most important meal of the day. Not only is it ideal for providing fuel for afternoon and evening activities, but if you recall the sequence of the Ayurvedic clock, with pitta is at the center of the day between 10 AM and 2 PM. It's when we are most productive and focused, but also when digestion is strongest, making it easier for us to break down food during this period, and decrease the risks of indigestion.

Digestion is always prioritized in Ayurveda, as it is believed that when we are unable to process and eliminate impeccably, we are left with an accumulation of undigested food, thoughts, emotions, and experiences, or *ama*. If you have ever uttered the phrase, "I need some time to digest this" in reference to thoughts or ideas, you understand that we process more than just food: We internalize, along with our meals, everything our eyes, ears, and mouth take in. Therefore, to make the healthful meals you prepare truly nourishing, consume them mindfully—with happy, friendly conversation or contemplative quiet. Given this information, you can conclude that the ubiquitous "sad-desk lunch" goes completely against the Ayurvedic grain—but so does the "working lunch," as lunch meetings are terrible for digestion and a prime opportunity to accumulate ama.

When ama begins to build, be it physical (like food) or emotional, it not only interferes with overall function, but also it settles into our vulnerable areas, making current symptoms worse and past conditions reappear. Thus, when you see ama on your tongue, be aware it could only be a short period of time before you start experiencing other ailments. Ama forms when there is low *agni*, or our main digestive fire. The commonality between digestion and fire is profound. Failure to feed a fire results in its burning out, and too much fuel will smother it. Our digestion is just the same: If we don't provide our body with food and something to burn, our metabolism will slow. If we overeat or become overstimulated, we will end up with more than we can efficiently process. Whether it be digestion of physical or mental food, an overtaxed digestion system never works properly.

Try this lunch meditation to feel the effects of truly digesting your food:

Transitioning into Evening

After lunch is the most common time for people to complain about being tired. It could be that an insufficient lunch isn't matching your energy needs, or perhaps you're simply overworked or under-rested. You'll find that no matter the cause, it's in our nature to look for instantaneous energy in something such as sugar or an afternoon coffee break. But what is genuinely rejuvenating is a restful break.

We know that the hours between 2 PM and 6 PM are vata time, meaning it's best to avoid food, drink, or activities that act as stimulants post-lunch. During this time frame, our internal clock is picking up its pace. Our reaction times are the quickest and our hand-eye coordination is also fast. Ingesting something else that amplifies this quickness will cause that energy to accumulate, and could result in the clichéd "3 PM slump."

What will bring balance to this state? As with most of Ayurveda's recommendations, attracting the opposite energy is key. Low energy requires a lift. Step outside for a leisurely walk, or just to take in some fresh air and daylight. Even on a cloudy day, the radiant sun can energize you in a ten-minute nature break. Or, practice meditation in a restorative yoga posture, such as lying on your back with your legs up the wall. Not only will this momentarily turn your world upside down, but also gravity will assist the flow of blood and lymph from your legs as a mild stimulation that helps you to feel lighter. Even pushing back from your desk and closing your eyes for a couple of minutes can give you a boost.

And since it's the time of day that our lung function is best, an afternoon breathing exercise (try *nadi shodhana*, page 167) could be the most invigorating option of all. Practice something you already know, or keep it simple by inhaling to a count of four and exhaling to a count of four, and repeating this for one to three minutes.

CHAPTER 6

Evening Rituals

Practices for Bringing Ease to the End of Your Day

atricharya is the practice of end-of-day rituals that cleanse the body and mind from all that's accumulated over the past several hours, and prepare us for the rest we need after a day full of activity. Many of the rituals are hygienic, ensuring that we've washed off the day and that our internal janitors can do their work while we sleep. A slow, relaxing evening full of these self-care routines can undoubtedly bring us quality, uninterrupted sleep—the foundation of good health and an established way to bring closure to a day or seasonal cycle. In honoring this gesture of completion, we are brought closer to our truest self and guided to our roles within nature.

Evening rituals and their representation of the end of a cycle play a special role in the prevention of accumulation. Without a nighttime pause, our experiences and ailments carry on from one day to the next. When there isn't respite from the anxiety you have about meeting a deadline, it will either interrupt your sleep or show up in your dreams. If you go to bed with the muscle tension that you felt in your shoulders while working on your computer all day, you'll probably wake up with it the next day, too. It can be difficult for our modern "push through it" society to see and accept, but the soft moonlight and stillness of the night is like a permission slip to wind down and take it easy. The yin—or lunar, feminine—qualities of an evening routine are something all of us could bear to embrace more.

The rituals provided here are aligned with Ayurveda's recommendation for closing out your day and setting you up for a restful night of sleep. Should you find you're still tossing and turning, or looking for the perfect herbal nightcap, refer to the rituals for insomnia on pages 215–20.

EAT A SMALL DINNER BEFORE 8 PM

Our body requires a generous window of time, at least two hours, between eating and sleeping for the night, so eating an early dinner is recommended. Also, since digestion begins to slow after 2 PM, dinner should be more of a tasting than a feast.

Western culture can make this ritual seem hard to adopt at first, since dinner has been deemed the hour for bonding and socializing. With the hectic schedules of children and adults alike, the entire family may not be home until 8 PM or later; by the time everyone has settled and dinner is on the table, it could be quite late and even overlapping with bedtime. And because dinner may be the only time that everyone sits together to catch up on one another's lives, more time and thought is put into it. This adds up to a bigger, home-cooked meal, typically serving as the centerpiece meal of the day. On the other hand, business and social meetings often take place over long, late-night dinners, which interrupts our digestion *and* sleep cycles (i.e., social jet lag from chapter 3).

But there's no need to eliminate the important ritual of family time, or times of quality bonding, to ensure healthy evening digestion, even if you're a family of one. You could still enjoy preparing and eating a well-rounded meal, but perhaps you eat less. If you've eaten an adequate lunch, there shouldn't be significant hunger this late in the day anyway. Portion out a small amount of what you make for dinner, savor it in the moment (remember your mindful eating practices from chapter 5), then package up the rest to take for lunch the next day. Ayurveda doesn't favor leftovers, because food loses its *prana* or energy the longer it is stored and the more times it is reheated. Yet, the remainder of a home-cooked meal will always win over food wrapped in plastic grabbed from a drive-through window; it will also keep you from skipping lunch entirely because nothing is conveniently available.

Dinner meals should also include food that is easier to digest, such as soup and well-cooked veggies. Heavier foods, like meat and dairy, will take longer to digest and might cause late-night indigestion that disrupts your sleep.

Implement a "no-glow rule" and shut off the things that emit blue light by 8 PM. Bonus points for shutting them down even sooner.

As discussed in chapter 3, blue light is interpreted in our brain as if it is daylight, which makes your body confused about which point in the twenty-four-hour cycle it is actually in. This could cause an improper or late release of melatonin, the hormone signaling your body that it is time for sleep, and disrupt your sleep cycles. If you find you must be on a device this late in the evening, turn it to a "night shift" mode that changes the light from cool to warm, or consider wearing glasses created to block blue light.

Wondering what to do without your tech? Read a book—a printed book that you can hold in your hands and turn the pages of. Try a short yoga practice or listen to music or a podcast. It isn't the best time for rock 'n' roll or an unsolved murder podcast, but rather something less stimulating, like classical music, ocean sounds, short stories, or a guided meditation. Think of other things that you like to do, such as journaling, drawing, knitting, or playing board games, and schedule them for this time of night.

RINSE YOUR BODY

Our primary bathing should be done in the morning; however, we should still take time to rinse our body of the dirt and debris we collected during the day before we go to bed. Rinsing in hot water may be too stimulating at night. If taking a shower, use lukewarm water and keep it brief. And if your favorite way to end the day is soaking in the tub, try using cooler water, placing a cool, damp cloth across your forehead, or bathing earlier in the evening. You could also forgo the shower and bath entirely and use a damp washcloth to wipe your body clean. At an absolute minimum, wash your face, hands, and feet.

WASH YOUR FACE

As is true for the body, oil cleansing is preferred over soap for the face because it can provide more nourishment to the skin. The skin on our face is more delicate than on our body and often has more exposure to environmental elements, so the gentle and soothing qualities of oil are especially appropriate. Since oil picks up particles of dirt, it can also effectively clean your skin without drying it out. As this approach has been adopted by modern skincare specialists, there are many oils that are marketed specifically for this use. You could select one of those, or start with plain jojoba, apricot kernel, or hemp seed oil from your *abhyanga* routine (see chapter 5).

Warm a small amount in your palms, then massage onto your skin. To remove the oil, use a warm, wet washcloth to dab or press onto your skin, repeating this until you feel the layer of oil is removed. You won't need much to hydrate your skin afterward. Our skin produces its own oil, or sebum, at night, and using more to moisturize can keep it from self-balancing. You might also find that a simple spritz of rose water will do the trick if you feel extra dry.

OIL YOUR HEAD

As we've seen, the soothing quality of oil makes it versatile in self-care practices. It is especially effective at easing the nervous system, hence its being a common Ayurvedic practice to use it to heal insomnia and facilitate deeper sleep.

Massaging oil all over the body, including the face, is one way to tap into this energy, but why not go right to the source—the top of your head? There are traditional Ayurvedic treatments to tap into the energetic, or *marma*, points in the head, but they require special equipment and trained practitioners. You can achieve a similar effect at home, however, with this simple nightly routine. Pour a quarter-size amount of sesame oil into your palm, or use an oil with herbs to promote restful sleep, such as lavender, passionflower, bhringaraj, valerian, and skullcap. Place it onto *adhipati marma*—the point that is considered to be the master of all marma. It is located at the small bump or peak at the crown of your head (called the posterior fontanelle); you can find this point by following the apex of each ear to the top of the head. Distribute the oil all over your entire scalp. Use the firm pressure of your fingertips, as you massage in a circular motion. For sleep, you may want to place a towel on your pillow so it does not get stained, despite this being a relatively small amount of oil.

OIL YOUR EARS

Karna purana, or ear oiling, is an evening ritual where warm oil is administered to the internal and external ear. Oiling your ears could preserve hearing and prevent hearing loss, reduce the frequency of ear infections, soothe ringing in your ears (tinnitus), or provide a general sense of grounding. As this can very temporarily muffle your hearing, it's recommended for the evening, when you can let the oil settle into your ears undisturbed.

Before bed, warm either sesame oil or an oil specifically formulated for ears. (If you have an ear condition, look for oils that contain garlic or mullein, two herbs that are used for reducing earaches and ear infections.) While lying on your side, drop three to five drops of oil into the upward-facing ear canal with a sterile dropper. You can increase this amount as you become more versed in the practice, and, of course, enlist the help of another if needed.

Once the oil is in your ear, press down on the the bump of cartilage in front of the ear (or tragus) and gently massage in a circular motion. Next, massage your outer ear in a gentle squeezing action. Then, gently hold your outer ear and carefully pull back, further helping to keep the oil in the ear canal and to open the eustachian tubes. Swallowing and yawning can also assist with this. Place a cotton ball in your ear before you turn over and treat the other ear, to prevent the oil from running out when you lie down.

OIL YOUR FEET

Nothing creates an immediate sense of grounding like rubbing oil into your feet. The heaviness of the oil and the dissolving of tension with massage makes it a magical antidote to a long day. And given the abundance of nerves and energetic connections between your feet and your entire body, this ritual is key to a night of sound sleep.

This practice involves very little effort and time compared to its significant benefits. Use a small amount of oil, about a dime-to-nickel-size amount for each foot, and apply it to your entire foot, including the top of each foot, soles, toes, and ankles. Once the oil is distributed, firmly massage the sole of each foot, paying special attention to your arches. Move to the top of each foot and make steady, longitudinal strokes between the bones. Then, massage each toe, ending with a gentle pull and a firm squeeze over each tip and the toenail. If you find an area that is particularly tense, give it special attention. When you are finished, slide on a pair of cotton socks to seal in the moisture and keep you from slipping.

As with all other methods involving oil, sesame is a go-to. If you find sesame has too strong or offensive a smell to be relaxing, another neutral oil, such as jojoba or grapeseed, will work nicely. You can also seek out oils that contain herbs or essential oils that help to calm and clear your mind. These can be the same oils you used on your head (see page 89).

CONSISTENTLY GO TO BED BY 10 PM

Putting your sleep times on repeat helps your body get the timing right for the entire day, enhacing your ability to stay consistent with all your rituals. You might find it hard to resist typical late-night activities at first, but your reward will be much greater: reliable rest. Showing up well-rested for your friends, family, and coworkers during the day will give you more quality time with them that they will appreciate!

By 10 PM, the time of transition from kapha to pitta, your body goes into restoration mode, making sure all systems are reset and that your natural cleansing and detoxification process (governed by pitta) is completed. But this only happens if you are asleep. If you stay awake, you'll be abusing your use of pitta. Many say they feel they have great focus or do their best work after 10 PM, and this is the reason why—that second wind of energy is your body going into pitta mode, and if you're not physically prepared for rest you could be kept up by it until the wee hours of the morning. All that fiery energy is redirected away from the liver and digestion, creating more likelihood of an *ama* buildup.

There's also something to be said about sleeping when the sun sleeps. As the sun sets long before 10 PM in the winter, you should be feeling the instinctive urge to go to bed earlier. We're designed to sleep when it is dark and play when it is light, so if it is dark longer, take nature's cue to indulge in more personal restoration.

Although we'd sometimes like to believe otherwise, restoration time can't be banked. If you miss a few hours of sleep during the week, sleeping longer on the weekend won't help. There's no such thing as procrastination when it comes to sleep. Staying up every now and then may be OK, but continued patterns of such can rob your body of its precious natural cleansing cycles.

SELF-STUDY

Slowing down at night balances out our tendency to push throughout the day. Do you make a conscious effort to bring peace and ease into your evening? How do you want your evenings to feel, and what mindful practices will you incorporate to help you arrive at this mental or emotional state?

CHAPTER 7

Seasonal Rituals

Practices for Changing with Nature

Aside from pulling out a favorite sweater, drinking hot cocoa, or adjusting the thermostat, not much about Western culture ritualizes seasons when it comes to health. By contrast, Ayurvedic texts offer detailed descriptions on seasonal changes and even give them a special name: *ritucharya*.

Like dinacharya and ratricharya, ritucharya is an outlined routine, though it is aligned with our calendar instead of our clock. Within its guidelines, we see the ways we should adjust our routine along with changes in climate, and how the timing between seasons—such as the spring and fall equinoxes, and winter and summer solstices—is the perfect time to focus on preventing illness. In addition to the seasons, there are other cycles that are longer than the twenty-four-hour clock, such as moon cycles. The full moon and new moon impact our physiology and create an energetic environment, making those phases the perfect time for rituals, self-reflection, and change.

Because the seasons differ in temperature and humidity, each season strongly relates to one dosha and its corresponding elements. Like we do in our personal constitutions, we try to maintain balance through the seasons by playing into the strengths of the elements, but also by seeking out pacifying actions. Everything in Ayurveda surrounds this idea. Doshas or elements can accumulate in the spring, summer, fall, and winter—a culprit behind seasonal illnesses. This can also be the cause for a deeper manifestation of an existing illness (for example, if you've had a fire or pitta imbalance brewing in the spring, it will be even worse in the fiery summer), or explain how you have an imbalance that isn't typical for your primary constitution (such as an earthy kapha person experiencing vata or air symptoms of dryness in the fall and early winter).

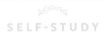

SELF-STUDY

Though we use the word *season* to describe weather changes and time periods throughout the year, the term is not limited to climate. As you read this chapter, also consider other phases, periods, or seasons that exist for you, such as the phases of your life, busy or slow seasons at work, and how you could use rituals and lifestyle modifications as you would for spring, summer, fall, and winter.

Excess of a quality, element, or dosha doesn't just cause an imbalance; it creates one that has similar qualities to the overabundant dosha. How would it feel to sit in the sun on a summer afternoon, donning a parka, while slurping spicy soup? What if you did this all season, and added on stressful work deadlines and a vigorous exercise schedule? Surely even the most enlightened among us would start to physically and mentally overheat. Indeed, hot summer often brings about conditions associated with heat, such as skin breakouts, inflammatory issues, and anger. With the dryness and lightness of fall and early winter, joint problems, constipation, dry skin, and insomnia rear their ugly heads. And in the dampness of spring, we come down with heavy, mucus-related conditions like allergies or early sinus infections.

Instead of our working against nature to fit our own needs and desires, Ayurveda teaches that when we accept what Earth provides, we keep seasonal illnesses at bay. If the season is dry, the produce that grows is naturally oily; if the climate is cool, the crops are heating. Thus, a pacifying routine aims to use things like seasonal foods, herbs, and spices as a primary source for maintaining balance.

Everything we consume has one or more taste associated with it, and this helps you to understand how what you eat affects you beyond its nutritional profile. Ayurveda recognizes six tastes: sweet, sour, salty, bitter, pungent, and astringent. These aren't always tastes you can identify on the tongue, but they are important when it comes to seasonal eating. What you'll learn throughout this chapter is what tastes dominate each season. In theory, the local farmers' market should double as your local pharmacy. In the chart below, note that (−) indicates a pacifying effect, and (+) indicates an aggravating effect.

Table 3. The Six Tastes

TASTES	ELEMENTS	DOSHIC EFFECT	PHYSIOLOGICAL EFFECTS	IF CONSUMED IN EXCESS	FOODS
Sweet	Earth + Water	V-P-K+	Builds and nourishes tissues, increases strength and vitality	Cough, congestion, diabetes, fatigue, heaviness, greed, laziness	Fruit, white rice, wheat, ghee, milk and cream, sweeteners
Sour	Earth + Fire	V-P+K+	Improves digestion by increasing salivation, energizing, cleansing	Hyperacidity, ulcers, rashes, eczema, acne, psoriasis	Fermented foods, yogurt, cheese, sour berries, citrus
Salty	Fire + Water	V-P+K+	Improves digestion by increasing salivation, digestion, absorption and elimination	Viscous blood, hypertension, skin conditions, water retention, edema, hyperacidity	Salt, seaweed or sea vegetables
Bitter	Ether + Air	V+P-K-	Detoxifying, decreases fevers, tones skin and muscle tissue	Dryness, dizziness, depletion, constipation	Leafy greens, dandelion, turmeric, neem, fenugreek, cacao, coffee
Pungent (spicy)	Air + Fire	V+P+K-	Clearing and cleansing, aids digestion, promotes absorption and elimination, improves circulation	Diarrhea, hyperacidity, ulcers, inflammatory skin conditions, excessive thirst	Garlic, onions, leeks, radishes, mustard greens and seeds, greens, peppers
Astringent (dry)	Air + Earth	V+P-K-	Stops bleeding, decreases sweating, reduces and tones tissues	Dryness, constipation, depletion, cramps	Cranberries, pomegranates, unripe bananas, beans, lentils, white potatoes, black tea, cruciferous vegetables

Daily routine activities and the types of exercise we partake in should naturally adjust with the seasons as well. Playing all day outside, as you did in the summer sun, just isn't as tantalizing—or possible—when the temperatures drop. When Earth becomes dormant, we follow her lead and spend more time indoors with books, soups, and board games. Then, just as we're getting cabin fever, she gives us the signs that it is time to blossom and breathe in the fresh air.

If you live in an area where there aren't distinct seasons of spring, summer, fall, and winter, you can still pick up on subtle changes in weather throughout the year. If it's still hard to define these shifts, you can adopt ritualistic changes at the mark of the spring and fall equinoxes and summer and winter solstices, which are also important times of change for our sun-based daily rituals. Our seasons, in fact, used to have even more definitive demarca-tions dividing them, but climate change has caused more extreme weather and blurred these boundaries.

SELF-STUDY

Using Table 3 as a reference, make a list of three foods or spices that you enjoy during each season. How do you feel when you eat these foods? Is there an emotional link to these tastes? Recognize these responses and how they not only associate with each season, but also how synchronized you are with nature when you eat them.

You'll find these seasonal rituals will be more like subtle alter-ations to your existing routines than new ones to implement. At the same time, remember that your family may have its own seasonal rituals, like a visit to the apple orchard, pumpkin patch, beach, or state fair, which are equally important to honor.

Late Winter and Spring (February–May)

The saying about April showers and May flowers is a tell-all for spring. There's a dampness and heaviness that accompanies the first months of the year, but what follows is a beautiful impulse to flower and grow.

Late winter and spring are considered to be kaphic months, or months that embrace the earth and water elements. This means it alternates between warm and cool, but is steadily heavy, wet, and stagnant feeling. If you can imagine, what happens in our body at this time is much like what happens with melting snow. By late winter, the snow accumulates—the dampness and coldness representing that of the kapha dosha. As the weather warms in the spring, the snow starts to melt, and in our body we experience this with feelings of stagnation, congestion, allergies, and excess mucus.

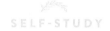

SELF-STUDY

Most of us either dread a change in the weather and activities, or look forward to them. The truth is, you can learn to love, and identify with, all of the seasons equally. Do you have a favorite season? If so, what makes it special? What season do you least enjoy? What traditions, routines, or rituals could help you make a better connection to that season?

What we need to combat all this moisture is light, dryness, and mobility.

And at this time of year, nature supplies us with just that: food that is light, astringent, and bitter as a counterbalance to her climate. Think of these qualities as you're making your shopping list. Fill your cart with sprouts, cruciferous veggies like broccoli and brussels sprouts, asparagus, berries, radishes, leeks, garlic, and leafy greens galore. Reduce intake of food that is heavier and oilier, like nuts or meat. If you are a meat eater, favor white meat or lighter fish.

Ayurveda will always favor eating cooked food, but spring, compared to fall and winter, is a more suitable time to incorporate some raw food into your diet. Try a bowl of fruit for breakfast or a small side salad as part of your lunch (not the whole meal). Incorporate spices that pack a pungent punch, such as pepper, garlic, ginger, cloves, and fenugreek.

After a full winter of rest, it's time to bring vigor back into your movement vocabulary. First, and foremost, it's important just to get moving. Find ways that you can add movement into your day, like walking after lunch. For your dedicated exercise, think sprints, interval training, and a program that overall leans toward cardio. Spring is associated with the kapha dosha, and so is the first cycle of life, from birth to puberty—which also represents a time of exploration and growth. Weave activities into your spring routine that have playful and childlike characteristics, and approach daily tasks as if they are brand new.

Begin the tradition of a spring ritual that embodies the concept of planting, new beginnings, and growth. Since spring has a natural momentum toward blooming, sort through the mundane areas of your life and find what needs a fresh start. Think of this time not only as spring cleaning for your home, but also spring cleaning for your personal intentions and goals.

Write down three things you wish to manifest this season and three words that describe your spring intentions. Breathing deeply, sit with your eyes closed to fully embody the newness spring will bring.

Summer (June–September)

Summer heat usually makes people either giddy or miserable, but no matter what tendency you fall toward there are practices that can make you feel more connected to this season.

With its abundance of daylight, summer is the season of fire, or the pitta dosha. *Sharp, light, hot, subtle,* and *oily* (or *dry* in excess) are all appropriate words to describe it. While chemically cooled air is a huge relief for overheating, incorporating cooler produce into your diet, along with calming breathing practices and more moderate exercise, is nature's preferred approach.

Summer bounty offers our bodies bitter, sweet, and astringent tastes, with summer squash, peas, celery, cucumbers, jicama, leafy greens, sweet berries, and herbs such as mint and cilantro.

Although you might crave cold beverages, continue to avoid ice in your drinks. Instead, sip on coconut water between your meals, which is not only a good way to defuse heat; it's almost like having an IV drip of electrolytes and hydration.

The physical activity you enjoyed in the spring should now slow and become more recreational; competitions and training goals can build too much heat. Swimming is the most pacifying activity for fiery times, but leisurely walks or bike rides can balance just the same.

Summer brings us time to sit back and unwind, but it's not all chill—research shows that crime increases in the summer. While the warm air may simply encourage lawbreakers to be out and about, this could also support the idea that summer heat can make us more vulnerable to pitta emotions, such as anger, frustration, and judgment. In addition to swapping out your food and exercise routine, try to be on the lookout for personal or professional encounters that involve heated discussions or get your blood boiling.

Just as the middle of the year is the pitta time of year, the middle of our life cycle is also a pitta time. From puberty to menopause, we are full of drive and aspirations that the fire element fuels in us. And as pitta is between birth and death, or between our beginning and ending, it is also the period of life that is about maintenance. So consider your summer practices to be like midlife: about sustaining and preserving.

Fall and Early Winter (October–January)

Whereas summer vibrates with high energy, fall and winter feel like the natural downshift. Playing into this vibe is exactly what you should do as the season trends toward vata dosha, or air and ether, and becomes light, dry, rough, hard, and mobile. Think of the dry leaves falling from the trees, or the cold and howling winter wind that makes you retreat indoors to sit by the fire.

The abundance of these qualities can lead to lost sleep, anxiety, constipation, and dry skin. Your instinct to reach for comfort (including foods) this time of year is the correct one—getting more rest, and enjoying warm drinks and heavier food is *not* counter to your fitness and desire to be productive in autumn.

The marketing whizzes at Starbucks may seem like geniuses for getting us to crave all things pumpkin and spice, but in reality they didn't have to work so hard. Our instinct to surround ourselves with cozy spices, whether in drinks, cooking, or scented candles, is in sync with nature's more subtle advertising. It's the time for nutmeg, cinnamon, allspice, ginger, and cardamom—all spices that pair well with our fall foods due to flavor, but also aid in processing the heavier harvest. They create warmth in the body after they are digested, and this, coupled with their ability to calm the nervous system, creates a cozy feeling from the inside out.

Mother Nature's food offerings have similar qualities. Here we find heavier, oily foods that doesn't spoil quickly, such as nuts, seeds, fall and winter squash, and the very food that anchors us with its name: root vegetables. Use them to prepare soups, stews, and porridge, which will warm your home and your being.

Rest is encouraged, but don't fall entirely off the exercise wagon. Adjust your movement practices to incorporate more strength training and endurance instead of focusing on intensity, intervals, or speed. Set your meditation timer for a longer duration and indulge in some slow, deep breathing (see ujjayi breathing on page 240).

In our lives, the end of the year genuinely feels like a time of closure. We close out business dealings, take time to celebrate holidays with family, and allow more time for rest before resolving to begin anew in January. We can reflect back on the fruits of our year-long laboring, the same way we harvest in the fall after a year of planting and growing. This is like our own life cycle on a smaller scale. As the last season of the year is represented by vata dosha, so too is the last season of life. After menopause and the male equivalent, or from retirement age onward, we are in the vata time of life. Similar to how in our later years, we feel a desire to slow down and take more time to enjoy life and recall happy memories, your urge to do the same every fall and winter is a natural one.

Finding order to your day is foundational and should always come before you tackle major changes in your diet, so that your digestive system can process what you eat. Not to mention, food lists can be quite overwhelming and difficult to follow. When you are ready to incorporate seasonal or doshic eating into your routine, use Table 4 as your guide. Note that some of the seasonal foods may come as a surprise to you, such as eating tomatoes in the fall or winter instead of the summer. This is because many foods are not native to our region and thus their harvest times have been modified to fit our climate. The foods fit with the season because of the balancing effects they have on our body.

Table 4. Seasonal Foods

Seasonal Eating: Late Winter to Spring, Kapha Dosha

Vegetables

Alfalfa Sprouts	Celery	Peas	Cranberries
Asparagus	Chili Peppers	Potatoes	Dried Fruit
Bean Sprouts	Collard Greens	Radishes	Lemons
Bell Peppers	Corn	Spinach	Limes
Broccoli	Fennel	Swiss Chard	Pomegranates
Brussels Sprouts	Green Beans	Turnips	Raspberries
Cabbage	Kale		Strawberries
Carrots	Lettuce	**Fruit**	
Cauliflower	Mustard Greens	Blackberries	**Meat and Fish**
	Onions	Blueberries	White Fish

Seasonal Eating: Summer, Pitta Dosha

Vegetables

Artichokes	Greens	Zucchini	Melon
Asparagus	Fennel		Pears
Beet Greens	Jicama	**Fruit**	Pineapple
Bell Peppers	Kale	Apples	Plums
Broccoli	Lettuce	Apricots	Pomegranates
Cabbage	Okra	Blueberries	Raspberries
Celery	Peas	Cherries	Strawberries
Cucumbers	Seaweed	Cranberries	**Meat and Fish**
Dandelion	Summer Squash	Grapes	White Fish
	Watercress	Guava	White Meat
		Mango	

Seasonal Eating: Fall to Late Winter, Vata Dosha

Vegetables

Avocado	**Fruit**	Peaches	Rice (Brown)
Beets	Bananas	Persimmons	Wheat
Brussels Sprouts	Dates	Tangerines	
Carrots	Figs		**Legumes**
Pumpkin	Grapefruit	**Meat and Fish**	Mung Beans
Winter Squash	Grapes	All Meat and	Tofu
Sweet Potatoes	Lemons	Fish	
Tomatoes	Limes		**Nuts and Seeds**
Turnips	Mango	**Grains**	Almonds
	Oranges	Amaranth	Brazil Nuts
	Papaya	Oats	Cashews
		Quinoa	Flaxseed

White Meat

Barley
Buckwheat
Millet

Kidney Beans
Lentils
Lima Beans

Mung Beans
Nuts and Seeds
Pumpkin Seeds
Sunflower Seeds

Ghee
Rice Milk

Corn Oil

Mustard Seed Oil

Black Pepper
Cardamom
Cayenne
Cilantro
Cloves
Fenugreek
Garlic

Ginger
Parsley

Honey
Molasses

Barley
Rice (white)
Legumes
Adzuki Beans
Fava Beans
Split Peas

Coconut

Flaxseed
Pumpkin Seeds
Sunflower Seeds

Coconut Milk
Cow's Milk
Ghee
Rice Milk
Soy Milk

Coconut
Olive
Soy
Sunflower

Cilantro
Coriander
Mint

Parsley
Saffron
Turmeric

Maple Syrup
Sucanat

Macadamias
Peanuts
Pecans
Pistachios
Walnuts

Butter
Buttermilk
Cheese

Ghee
Kefir
Yogurt
All Nut and Seed
Milks

Avocado
Ghee
Sesame

Anise
Asafoetida (Hing)
Basil
Cardamom
Cumin
Garlic
Ginger
Rosemary

Sage
Thyme
Turmeric

Honey
Molasses

Seasonal Transitions

Our seasonal rituals can be carefully placed within their designated months, but there are also rituals reserved for when seasons connect. The merging of the seasons is called *ritusandhi,* which means the joint between the seasons. Similar to how we earlier discussed the afternoon being a crucial time to pause and take inventory of how we feel, this, too, is a transitional time that deserves its own practices.

Ritusandhi covers an approximately two-week period that marks the end of one season and the start of another. The two equinoxes and two solstices are traditional landmarks for these times; however, climate changes have made those dates on the calendar less reliable. Even if you can't feel a change, you can approximate your area's ritusandhi with the more consistent rise or fall in temperatures or humidity. Though a random hot or cold day (or week) could occur, you feel as though the season has set in.

This is the most customary time to do a mental and physical reset, unless you are performing a cleanse for other purposes. This signals our body for what is yet to come, while simultaneously making up for any properties that may have accumulated prior. Once held by the definitive properties of spring, summer, fall, or winter, we have a vulnerability between the seasons that our transitional routines can cushion.

For those living geographically where there are four seasons, you may be more fully aware of your tendency toward seasonal illnesses that happen every fall or spring, but also the between-season illnesses that happen as the weather is shifting. The familiar scene goes a little something like this: The dry fall air moves in and you start to experience categorically dry conditions; you might get joint aches, constipation, dry skin, dry sinuses, or an occasional cough, cold, or sore throat. Not knowing that you could have avoided these periodic imbalances with transitional routines, or modified practices during the season, the illnesses go without remedy. The dryness accumulates throughout the winter, but once your body decides it's had enough, its innate intelligence kicks in and begins producing more mucus, or causing itself to retain fluid to balance the dryness. But by the time that happens, the moist and heavy winter air of spring is already making its way in. As this meets your body's own attempt to balance with moisture of its own, you start to experience allergies and conditions related to an overproduction of mucus. It's a never-ending cycle, tiring to even read about!

No matter how impeccable our routine is during each season, there is still a risk of accumulation and a need to change our practices for the upcoming season. One way to go about this is with a seasonal reset or a ritusandhi cleanse. This provides the time, space, and energy for

SELF-STUDY

Are there times of year when you are predictably sick? Is it usually with the same illness? Do these times match nature's seasons, or a personal season, such as work or school? Consider your seasonal practices and determine what could change (food, sleep, exercise, etc.) to help your immunity weather the effects.

digesting the experiences, food, and emotions that occurred during the previous months.

Ayurveda's traditional between-season reset is called *panchakarma*, which means "five actions." Panchakarma is a purification process that is performed periodically, but is also used as a precursor to medicinal treatment. The five components:

- *nasya*—herbs administered through nose;
- *vamana*—therapeutic vomiting;
- *virechana*—purgation or laxative therapy;
- *basti*—enema therapy; and
- *rakta moksha*—bloodletting.

Together, they act to clear the body and mind of anything that might hinder the action of any medicines that are taken. It can be thought of as rinsing and wringing out a sponge so that it is free to fully absorb once again. In its entirety, this is a very lengthy and involved process that should only be performed under supervision, but there are abbreviated versions of Ayurvedic cleanses that can be done on your own.

Whether you choose to go to a center or conduct your own reset at home, *kitchari* will always be a part of it. Kitchari is a porridge-like dish made of mung beans and white basmati rice, along with delicious spices that specially heal digestion. It can include cooked vegetables that appease your dosha, imbalance, or season. Chutneys, or herbal sauces or jams, can also be used to make kitchari more dosha specific. But even just on its own, by Ayurvedic standards it's the most nourishing food one can have. It supports the body's natural cleansing system without deprivation, as the beans and rice together make a complete protein we can easily digest.

A basic, but beneficial, at-home cleanse is a kitchari mono-diet. For three to five days, for breakfast, lunch, and dinner, you eat kitchari. In between meals, you drink warm water or digestive teas, like cumin, coriander, and fennel tea (CCFT) (see pages 199–200). The idea is to be easy on the digestive system, but you'll be surprised at how it also lightens your mental load: Not having to plan your meals frees up a lot of headspace for mental processing. You can increase the effectiveness of your cleanse by adding more time for self-care through things like daily massage, yoga, breathing exercises, meditation, and journaling. Though you should always consult with your healthcare practitioner, this short version is safe for almost everyone.

Healing Kitchari Recipe

Makes 12 cups (2L) or 6 servings

> 1 cup (175 g) white basmati rice
>
> 1 cup (200 g) yellow mung beans (soaked overnight)
>
> 1 tablespoon ghee or coconut oil
>
> 2 teaspoons mustard seeds
>
> 1 inch (2.5 cm) ginger root, peeled and minced
>
> 2 tablespoons ground cumin
>
> 1 teaspoon ground turmeric
>
> 1 bay leaf

recipe continues

1 teaspoon salt

2 cups (300 g) chopped seasonal vegetables (optional)

Doshic- or seasonal-specific chutneys (optional)

1. Rinse the rice and the soaked mung beans until the water runs clear.

2. Heat the ghee or oil in a large pot over medium heat. Add the mustard seeds and slowly stir until you hear the first mustard seed pop. Immediately add the ginger, cumin, turmeric, bay leaf, and salt. Stir slowly for 30 seconds to 1 minute.

3. Add the rice and mung beans to the pot and stir until the oil and spices are distributed evenly. Add 6 cups (1.5 L) water and bring to a boil. Reduce to a simmer and cover.

4. Cook, stirring occasionally, for about 45 minutes, or until the rice and mung beans are soft and the water has fully absorbed. If you're adding root vegetables or longer-cooking veggies, add them about 20 minutes into cooking. Toss in any leafy greens about 10 minutes before the end of the cook time. The mung beans may start to break apart. If the mixture becomes too dry or starts sticking to the bottom before it is fully cooked, add more water.

5. To serve, optionally add a spoonful of chutney, top sesame seeds, cilantro, or parsley, if using.

Vata or Fall and Early Winter Chutney

Makes 2 cups (300 g)

1 cup (150 g) raisins

1 cup (100 g) dates, pitted and chopped

1½ teaspoons ground cumin

½ teaspoon ground cardamom

½ inch (1 cm) fresh ginger, peeled and minced

1 tablespoon fresh orange juice

Pinch of salt

1. Soak the raisins and dates in enough room-temperature water to cover for 10 minutes.
2. Drain the water and add the raisins and dates to a food processor or blender.
3. Add the cumin, cardamom, ginger, orange juice, and salt and pulse or blend until the mixture is a jam-like texture. Store refrigerated in an airtight container for up to two weeks.

Pitta or Summer Chutney

Makes 2 cups (300 g)

¾ cup (75 g) shredded unsweetened coconut

1½ cups (35 g) fresh mint leaves

Juice of one lime

2 teaspoons maple syrup

Pinch of salt

Add the coconut, mint, lime juice, maple syrup, and salt to a food processor or blender. Pulse or blend to combine the ingredients. Water may be added, 1 tablespoon at a time, until the mixture is a thick puree. Store refrigerated in an airtight container for up to one week.

Kapha or Late Winter and Spring Chutney

Makes 1 cup (150 g)

2 cups (50 g) fresh cilantro

1 inch (2.5 cm) fresh ginger, peeled and minced

recipe continues

1 medium-size green chili, approximately ¼ cup (50 g) chopped (use more or less depending on spice preference)

1 tablespoon fresh lime juice

Pinch of salt

1. Wash the cilantro, remove the stems, and coarsely chop the leaves.
2. Add the cilantro leaves, ginger, chili, lime juice, and salt to a food processor or blender.
3. Pulse or blend until you have created a puree. Water may be added, 1 tablespoon at a time, until the mixture has reached the desired consistency. Store refrigerated in an airtight container for up to one week.

Moon Cycles

The moon has an impact on the ocean's tide, animal behavior, human physiology, and our ability to manifest dreams right into reality. The lunar cycle is twenty-nine and a half days long, and its undeniable potency has made the moon a keystone of ceremonies, traditions, and practices within different cultures. While there are a fair amount of myths and legends surrounding the moon, there is an equal amount of research being conducted to find a correlation behind the cycles of the moon and the cycles of living things.

From learning the best time to plant or harvest, to having a better understanding of melatonin release, to uncovering more about the timing of female reproductive cycles, a lot has been discovered about what happens during the waxing and waning phases of the moon. If we take even a small portion of what we know and apply it to the way we conduct our lives, we will be one step closer to having conscious connection with nature.

Creating rituals to honor the new and full moon is a powerful way to celebrate earth's sacred satellite, and we don't have to believe the moon is mystical or magical to do so. It is no different than answering the sun's invitation to be active in work or play, to recognize the moon's signals to pause and slow down at times we might otherwise plunge through.

NEW MOON RITUAL

The new moon is the first phase of a moon cycle. Within our physiology, it is most commonly the time for female menstruation and when the most melatonin, the hormone regulating circadian rhythm, is released. For those gardening with the moon cycles, this is an optimal time for planting seeds. Overall, this phase represents a time of growth and renewal, making it a wonderful time to dream, wish, and set goals. This new moon ritual is meant for guiding you through such a process.

Create a sacred space.
Find a quiet space in your home or outside. Allow it to be clear of clutter and distractions, but let it be home to the sacred things you adore, such as plants, candles, crystals, or photos of people who love and inspire you. This can be a temporary setup, since it could take some time to determine the best place and elements you need to make it special. But as the months go by and these rituals become more routine for you, you might be inspired to make it a permanent fixture. When you get to that point and

decide on the perfect arrangement, be invested in its upkeep—clean and revive it energetically with fresh flowers, or rearrange it with each moon cycle or season so that it doesn't become energetically stagnant. It can become the nesting ground for daily or nightly rituals, including your meditation practice or journaling. Furthermore, consider ringing a bell or chime or lighting incense or sage to help clear the space with each use. This will signify that something special is about to begin.

HOW TO CREATE YOUR HOME ALTAR

Having a dedicated place in your home that represents what is important in your life can be the perfect reminder to slow down and add more mindful moments to your day. Though they can be a place for prayer, altars need not be reserved for religious use. Rather, an altar is an external reminder of the people and values you hold dear. Start by finding a place in your home that is clear of clutter. It is nice to have a location that is somewhat removed from the main action of your family, but at the same time, somewhere you will see it often. Use a small table or a shelf, and choose photos, art, or journals to place upon it. Consider things to represent the different elements of nature, such as stones, flowers, a small mirror to represent water, or a candle to represent fire. Only select the things that are meaningful to you, instead of trying to fill the space. Leave room for anything you may want to add in time, and be open to the idea of changing items as your needs change.

Repeat a mantra, affirmation, or prayer.

Take an intentional seat, an upright position that feels supported without being rigid and allows you to breathe freely with ease. Choose a phrase associated with creating, openness, and readiness to help align you with the intention you seek for this new moon, such as "I am prepared and equipped for what is yet to come." You can read the mantra aloud, repeat it to yourself silently, or write it down—as long as you give it some kind of voice, it doesn't matter who hears it (or doesn't).

Make a list of five intentions.

Write down your intentions, or things you'd like to manifest, using "I" statements: "I am" or "I will." It's important to put the pen to paper using your voice. The tactile experience of writing makes your statements feel more real and provides you with a physical list you can eventually hold or place in a sacred space.

Meditate.

Take at least five to ten minutes to sit comfortably, with your eyes closed, visualizing the actualization of each item on your list. When you are done, place your list somewhere you will see it often, such as your bedside table or an altar in your sacred space. Allow it to serve as a reminder for the things you will manifest with this new moon.

FULL MOON RITUAL

The full moon is considered to be a most auspicious time. Just as the gravitational pull of the moon can draw upon the ocean tide, it is said to draw out the essence of plants and medicine. For this reason, Ayurvedic tradition considers it the best time to make ghee, since the essence of the juice and milk used to make it is enhanced during this lunar period.

This ability of the full moon to draw out also makes it a good time for us to intentionally release what we no longer need. This full moon ritual can be used to facilitate the process of letting go.

Create and clear your sacred space.

Similar to how you established a space with the new moon, you'll choose either a spot next to your altar or another quiet place in your home or in nature to conduct your full moon ritual. Items you have in this area should feel comforting and supportive. Palo santo, also called holy wood, or sage can be burned to energetically clear your space.

Repeat a mantra, affirmation, or prayer.

Create a statement or phrase that you can write or say aloud or to yourself that invokes a liberating energy, such as, "I let go of what is no longer of benefit to me." Calling up forgiveness and release will help align you with the process of freeing yourself of things that have been accumulating and hindering you in the previous cycle.

Write a list of three things you wish to release.

Recognize patterns in your life that are no longer of service or that may be abusing precious energy or *prana*, and think about how you may replace them with a new intention or ritual. Using these things as a guide, write an "I" statement of release for each, such as, "With this full moon I release _____ and welcome the ability to _____."

Place your list on your altar or in a special place.
Choose a sacred space to place your written statements, either together with or separate from your new moon intentions. Pause for several deep breaths before them, feeling the weight of each element to be let go being lifted from your chest and shoulders, allowing you to breathe deeper.

PART 3

The Foundations
for
Ritual Success

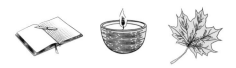

CHAPTER 8

Your Pranic Budget

Allocating Your Energy to What Matters Most

We flourish in the areas of our life where we direct our energy. When we feel unfulfilled or unhappy, we might recognize the need for change, but wrapped up in our current situation and storyline, it's challenging to see what parts of our lives are working for us, and what is not. This is especially true if you're in a career that you love and participating in other activities you feel passionate about, but still feel off—why put in extra energy to change what is supposedly feeding your desire for life?

Prana is a Sanskrit word that means "life force," and can also be translated to "breath." When we eat food that is high in prana and have relationships and tasks we enjoy, we feel energized. Being filled with prana makes us vibrant and happy. But engaging in activites that are mundane, mindless, or uninteresting can drain us of prana. Without taking a moment to evaluate where we are directing our energy, we become at risk of a pranic leak, oblivious to life force that is slowly trickling away.

It's ideal to be saving more prana than you are spending. This exercise will help you determine the sustainability of your current routine by balancing your pranic budget. Take a glimpse at which parts of your life perhaps cost more than they give back, or vice versa. In doing so, you'll see how you can redirect your energy to balance your books perfectly. Consider doing this as you feel it's necessary, but also check in periodically throughout the year, such as at the beginning of a new season as a way to honor the natural shift in energy.

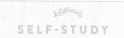

SELF-STUDY

At a glance, what are some of the daily sources of "leaky prana," such as small talk, gossip, checking your phone, or worrying about the past? What techniques could you use to become more aware of this and to stop the leak?

1. Determine and eliminate the unnecessary

Create a list of tasks, activities, and to-dos that occur for you on an average day. Though it could feel tedious and nitpicky to go through every single thing you do on any given day, it's important to note what is most consistent and what consumes the most time. If you prefer, you can create two lists for work and home life. Additionally, you can create a separate list for weekly and monthly tasks.

Some things may be necessary, but others may not be—or perhaps they're things that you're no longer giving 100 percent to or feeling fully committed to. Next to each task, write "N" (for *necessary*) or "U" (for *unnecessary*) to indicate its importance.

Example:

Grocery shopping: N

Emails: N

Accounting: N

Volunteering: U, but feel contribution to society

Massage appointment: N, allows for stress relief and physical well-being

Weekly professional networking: U, but contributes to business growth

Next, go through each item and mark a positive (+) if they fuel you or a negative (−) or if they deplete or drain you. Scale the effect from 1 to 3, 1 being a small effect on your energy that you can tolerate, and 3 being a high effect. Then, tally your energy balance.

Example:

Grocery shopping: N (−1)

Emails: N (−3)

Accounting: N (−1)

Volunteering : U, but feel contribution to society (+2)

Massage appointment: N (+3)

Weekly professional networking: U, but contributes to business growth (−2)

Overall energy balance = (−2)

2. Make a plan for acceptance or change

Looking at your list, do you now realize how certain tasks are depleting, and while maybe they felt necessary, they actually weren't? Cross off the items you can officially do without and map out a plan to change, delegate, or eliminate that activity as needed. Having a timeline for this change could serve as a motivator.

It would be unrealistic to expect that we can remove all the things in our lives that deplete us; many of them are just necessary for our day-to-day livelihood. For each of these items on your list, create a plan for acceptance or change of perspective. Consider small changes you could make to the routine that would give it more pranic value: turning on some music while doing laundry, going to a café to catch up on email, or bringing a friend along to the grocery store can make a big difference.

Example:

Grocery shopping: N (–1)

Plan for change: Subscribe to a weekly online grocery shopping and delivery service to both plan ahead and ensure that all the staple items for the week will be stocked at home. Make the more spontaneous trips for fresh ingredients when I am already out or on my way home from work.

Emails: N (–3)

Plan for change: Create different mailboxes so that messages can be organized by both priority and subject matter. Rather than checking email consistently throughout the day when it can't consciously be tended to, spend the morning replying to email and the evening organizing and delegating.

Accounting: N (–1)

> **Plan for change:** Choose one day a week when accounting will take place. Go to my favorite coffee shop to complete the task so that there is a more exciting feel to this mundane task.

Volunteering: U, but feel contribution to society (+2)

> **Plan for change:** Discontinue volunteering in two weeks; reconsider when I have more time and energy.

Massage appointment: N (+3)

> **Plan for change:** Continue to make massage a priority. Schedule next 3 monthly appointments now, so that I don't have an excuse to skip.

Weekly professional networking: U, but contributes to business growth (–2)

> **Plan for change:** Reduce to monthly. After two months, evaluate to see if growth was impacted by reduced attendance. If no negative impact, discontinue entirely. If it was impacted, ask a friend to join me each week to make it more appealing.

3. Plan to refuel

After two weeks, check in on how your plans are going. Where have you been falling off course? Are there things you would love to do that aren't on your daily list or aren't being prioritized? Many times we can bring life to these tasks by making them a constant in our daily rituals and routines. Write out what some of the things that fuel you are and devise a plan for making them a bigger part of your life.

Example:

Going for bike rides: Sunday afternoons are times when I don't have much focus and begin to dread the week ahead. Going for a bike ride at this time would be encouraging and motivating.

Reading: Instead of zoning out to Netflix on the couch at night, I will select three books from my bookshelf and commit to reading three nights a week to finish them.

Travel: I'll block my calendar so that I can have a three-day weekend for a mini-getaway every month.

CHAPTER 9

Keeping Course

Common Obstacles and Tips for Overcoming Them

As much as it may hurt, we often learn best from our mistakes, letting each experience inform the next. This is why being aware of potential obstacles and what to do when you encounter them helps when establishing new rituals. Still, it sure does feel good when the right amount of preparation results in smooth sailing, so it's equally important to plan ahead for what will help you succeed directly. Restructuring how you spend your days isn't easy for anyone, of any constitution, so consider these tips for helping you find success in being consistent with your rituals.

Be Aware of Potential Obstacles

Your concerns, excuses, and reasons could be legitimate, false, or premature, but it doesn't matter in the end. In your world, they exist. Having foresight into the issue is invaluable and will leave you prepared and equipped for what's to come.

1. IF YOU DON'T KNOW WHAT TO DO OR WHERE TO BEGIN . . .

"Start simple" and "simply start" are two mantras that reiterate how the basics are enough. If you are waiting for the perfect moment or until you feel like you are absolutely ready to begin, you might never start. Decipher if what you're perceiving as uncertainty about rituals—which ones to try, how to do them, when to fit them in—is really just a way to delay change. If you decide you're hesitant to change, refer back to chapter 2, where we identified the need for change, or chapter 4, where we discussed how our doshas react to rituals and routine. Review the chapter self-study questions to recognize potential patterns in delaying change, or even remember times where you waited so long to feel ready that you let an opportunity pass. If, alas, it turns out you're truly lost on where to begin, here's what you can do.

Start with what you've discovered about yourself thus far. Choose a specific area of your life or aspect of your well-being that needs to be addressed, or choose a time of day, such as when you consistently feel tired, least focused, or have never really had a good vibe. Think about daily activities that you might add to those areas or times to bring you joy and align with your needs. This is a perfect opportunity to integrate a new ritual and may leave you looking forward to these times rather than dreading them.

2. IF YOU'RE TOO TIRED AND CAN'T SPARE THE EXTRA TIME OR MONEY FOR SELF-CARE . . .

Getting up earlier, staying up later, or mustering extra time and energy for self-care may not feel possible with your lifestyle right now. But adding insult to injury is the fact that these overwhelmed times are usually when we need it most. If the mere thought of adding something minimal, like drinking lemon water, to your morning rituals exhausts you, increasing the components of your routine isn't the answer. What you need is a personal reorganization.

Your path is going to be cleared by delegating extraneous tasks, optimizing your planning, and putting systems in place. Start by assessing the less-vital things on your daily checklist that could be delegated to someone else, or be set aside to complete at another time. Could a family member act as your sous chef? Are there coworkers you could partner with to alternate bringing a fresh, home-cooked lunch to the office to share? Do you have an assistant at work who could reply to simple emails? If not, could you hire an assistant? Is it vital that everything on your list be done right now? Contemplate possibilities that are outside of your usual solutions.

The idea of a personal reorganization can be very overwhelming, especially for the vata dosha which can be easily distracted and overwhelmed. There can be temptation to cling to tasks because you feel like you need to control them yourself or because you have always done them is an energy suck. Kaphas get stuck in this cycle because they would rather keep things the way they are, and we know that pittas struggle with a need to control, but it can be liberating to have help. It's true that no one else will do something just the way you would, and to your standards, but having tasks completed frees up precious time that can now be dedicated to your personal care and healing. Weigh the importance of your health against things being up to snuff. We are talking about your well-being, after all. Plus, nothing is permanent, so once you have your self-care systems in place, you can reevaluate if there are things that really should only be done by you.

Finally, find other areas where systems could be in place. Think about this as automatic bill-pay for your life. Most people generally eat the same foods or at least use the same staple ingredients during a week's time. What about having those staple groceries delivered once a week so that there are fewer last-minute trips to the store for things you need to feel well? The same goes for your toiletries. You probably can predict when you're going to need a new bottle of shampoo or a roll of toilet paper. Can there be a scheduled day for this type of shopping each month, or what about subscription services or companies that provide autorefill for everyday items? When these needs are automatically being met, you can think less about supplying your self-care and have more time to just do it. All of your preparation, delegation, and systemization clears your headspace and direct your energy to enjoying your wellness rituals.

If you're reading this and worrying about when you'll find time to make schedules for toilet paper runs or daily to-do lists for your assistant, consider this: The dedicated, one-time, hour or more session it takes to get some of these methods in place will spare you extra minutes and hours going forward *every day*. And if you don't feel like you even have this amount of time to plan, know that you can create a change with the smallest increments. The idea isn't to fill every minute of your day, so look for times where there are already transitions or natural pauses and cherish them. You could stretch when you get up from your chair or practice a two-to-three-minute breathing exercise before you head off to lunch—the little things add up. Do what you can and remember that the accumulative effect of consistency is key. You'll be giving your nervous system room to breathe—and a boost in energy shortly after.

3. IF YOUR DAYS ARE TOO UNPREDICTABLE FOR PLANNING, OR THE RESPONSIBILITIES OF EACH DAY FLUCTUATE BASED ON WORK REQUIREMENTS OR FAMILY AND PERSONAL NEEDS . . .

The details of all of our days are always changing, never quite the same—we wear different things, encounter different people as we go to and fro, and of course feel differently, even with the best routines in place. For some, though, the circumstances of where you live, the hours you work, or the tasks required to care for relationships and family may make it seem like each day is radically different from the day before. If this is you, there is always something that you can make happen at the same time each day. Could one meal be a recurring event? Perhaps it isn't possible to go to bed at the same time every night, but could you have the same routine before you go to bed? Could you have the same wake-up time to complete at least half a consistent cycle? How about stepping outside for a breath of fresh air when the clock strikes 3 PM every afternoon? Begin with what is possible, and what you feel would be most nourishing.

If even these small choices seem out of your control—your 3 to 4 PM could be all yours one day, but a client's another day and your baby's the next—consider the notion that you may actually be able to streamline more than you think possible. Is the unpredictability of your day on your shoulders, or are you too readily meeting the needs of a role someone else has asked you to play? Could your business call happen outside instead of in front of a computer, or your parenting time take place on a leisurely stroll instead of on the couch? Sometimes we submit ourselves to the idea that there isn't another way, even without self-inquiry or asking others for help. Instead of assuming that you can't take your lunch at the same time each day, discuss the importance of it with your boss. It could be that nobody has ever asked to do it differently. People generally want to help other people and to be as supportive of you as they can.

If you are self-employed or are able to create your own schedule to some degree, your argument for lack of control weakens. It becomes more a question of what and, more important, *who* you are prioritizing. Put yourself first and opt to give yourself the healthy structure you deserve. You'll be able to show up better for others because of it.

When it absolutely, unequivocally isn't possible to allocate one time to one specific agenda, do your best to create a comforting ritual around an activity and to perform it with as much mindfulness as possible. To those of you working night shifts, this one is especially beneficial for you. For example, if you can't have breakfast at the same time every day, let the eating process be methodical whenever it happens, such as with the lunch meditation on page 82. Place your plate or bowl in front of you. Close your eyes to take several deep breaths and to consider the source of your nourishment. Then, continue to eat without performing any other activity.

4. IF YOU LIVE WITH OTHER PEOPLE WHO ARE ON DIFFERENT SCHEDULES WITH DIFFERENT AGENDAS . . .

This can be one of the most difficult obstacles to creating routines, especially if you are the caregiver for people whose schedules or agendas conflict with yours.

Sharing a living space can present a challenge when it comes to coordinating eating and sleeping times. You could be the one waking up early, moving stealthily through the house so that nobody else wakes, imbuing your rituals with stress and fear of waking up the others. Or maybe you're the one trying to get to bed early, but you have to deal with someone rolling into bed or jolting you awake with outside noises hours after you've been asleep. Whatever the scenario, it's likely easily solved with a little love and understanding. Outline to your space-mate how you've been feeling, how your proposed changes will make you feel better, and—the key point—tell them how your feeling better will also be beneficial for them. Most people want to surround themselves with happy people and want those they love to be receiving the nurturing they need, even when needs differ. You may find yourself making some compromises, but providing a clear explanation of what you need is the first step in forming a schedule ally.

When you're at the mercy of a different person's agenda because you provide care for them, the solution is most often to enlist help. If you don't, your resources for giving will be exhausted, much like pitta overload that comes from overworking or working late into the night. Ask friends, neighbors, or family members if they can "cover" for you for an afternoon or an entire day. It doesn't even need to be a regular commitment—even one day a month will be twenty-four entire hours you have free to dedicate to self-care. Remember: A self-care day isn't necessarily a (potentially expensive) spa day; it can just be a day without goals or expectations, aside from your long-term goal of feeling well.

As with all our self-care planning, a bit of time and foresight will help prevent your agenda-free days from being stressful. Take out your calendar and block out daily, weekly, bimonthly, or monthly "ojas days," or time frames that you can commit to for restoring your energy, just as you commit to helping others the rest of the time. *Ojas* is an Ayurvedic term that means vitality, immunity, or health reserves. It's what you call upon when you feel you are becoming ill and don't have the energy you need to ward off sickness. If you've been traveling and are run down, having strong ojas will keep you well. Unlike with restorative time itself, you can stockpile ojas. You can do this with specific food and herbs, like ghee, shatavari, ashwagandha and dates (see chapter 11 for more suggestions), but you can also build ojas by doing things you love and by being with the people you adore most. So make these your "no goal days"—or rather, a day where the only goal is to feed your soul with what it hungers for.

Tips for Staying on Track

1. BE CONSCIOUS OF TIME AND SPACE

One of the worst feelings is when something goes wrong and you don't have the time to manage it. And if we're being honest, isn't that typically *when* things go wrong? It could be as simple as a coffee spill on your shirt before a big meeting or date, or something more complex, like having to repair foundation damage to your house after a flood. There's also those times when we feel too tired to do anything extra, even if it is taking only a few minutes to brush your teeth or wash your face before bed. When there isn't wiggle room, panic ensues, or we neglect taking even small amounts of time for better self-care.

When planning out your new routine, be sure to leave space for the unknown. Estimate the amount of time you need to mindfully conduct each part of your ritual, then schedule yourself for more time than you actually need, or think you'll need. Many of the most transformative rituals (like oiling your feet at night) are not a huge time commitment, but having a buffer could be what actually allows you to carry out what you intend. Plan ten minutes for a five-minute morning meditation practice, so if you need extra time to settle into your quiet space it's available. Pencil in fifteen minutes more than you really need for eating your lunch. This way you won't have to rush through it or skip it entirely if you get held up. Giving yourself space not only allows you to feel calm and present no matter what shows up, but also it can be encouraging when you feel unmotivated. When you realize that you could feel better without the huge time commitment, you're more likely to be consistent.

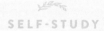

SELF-STUDY

In looking at your schedule, when do you envision your rituals taking place? What is a small but realistic amount of time that you can devote to self-care and healthy routine without the task being daunting or causing strain?

2. ASK FOR SUPPORT AND AIM FOR ACCOUNTABILITY

For a ritual to be effective and consistent, you may need someone or something to hold you accountable. Know yourself and what would normally work for you, as well as *who* you choose to help. Do you need to announce it to your whole office, to family, or on social media? Or do you prefer things more intimate, like asking a partner or best friend to share the ritual with you and be a lifeline when you need help? Or is it more effective for you to keep things private, with a tracking app, a journal, or a chart? Being honest with yourself about what keeps you committed and reliable will keep you more accountable.

Accountability is paramount in keeping your expectations realistic and suitable for you. If you keep having to report to your allies that you missed your morning yoga practice, they can help you identify your area of weakness: Maybe you are trying to do too many new things at once, or maybe trying to squeeze yoga into a busy morning isn't as feasible as practicing at night. Without someone to check in with, you might instead push through and feel defeated by rituals in general, rather than having those set times and people to help you identify a small detail that might be tweaked and therefore lead to success.

Education and perspective are also key; people can't easily see things from your side if they don't understand the meaning behind it. You may find that your commitment to being of healthier body and mind can be isolating. The looks you get when asking for water without ice in a restaurant or eating kitchari in a breakroom filled with people eating take-out or pre-packaged lunches can be a deterrent. Let people into the ritual club by explaining your practices and why they're important to your well-being. Your friends, space-mates, or coworkers may eventually want to adopt some rituals themselves if they identify with your reasoning. At the very least, if they're not interested in doing these things for themselves, they might be able to hold you accountable. Without being commanding, be specific about the ways that they can assist you in reaching your goal. When you include people and make them a part of the process, they are even happier when they see your success.

3. MAKE SEASONAL CHANGES OR MODIFICATIONS FOR HOW YOU FEEL

There may be some exceptions, but most people's needs will change throughout the year and throughout their lives. This is because of our connection to nature, internally and externally. In addition, the effectiveness of your routine can be called into question if you've never modified it. Think about your favorite shirt—you may love wearing it and how it makes you feel, but eventually it will wear out and no longer serve you in the way it once did. To continue wearing it might make you feel worse, instead of better about how you look and feel.

A very natural way to go about this is to change your routine with the seasons. "Seasonal" in this case could refer to either climate changes associated with the time of year (as we discussed in chapter 7) or the work climate that is associated with your company's busy season. For tax accountants, your self-care routine should change as April 15 nears, because prepping other people's taxes won't give you the same amount of time to prep for your own wellness. Or if you're a wedding photographer, it would only be natural to modify your health rituals during the busy wedding months of May and June. Such changes can be as simple as swapping out an ingredient in your meals to optimize digestion, or practicing more vigorous movement in the spring and more grounding movement in the fall and winter as you need. It could mean adding or taking away from what you currently do, omitting one element of a routine to keep you from avoiding it entirely when you find yourself continually strapped for time. Our need for balance is unabating, but what we need is variable. Without letting yourself obsess or overanalyze, be informed as to what will serve you in the present.

4. BE REALISTIC, SIMPLISTIC, AND CONSISTENT

Even if you're an "all or nothing" type of person, small changes are recommended. Just because you think you can handle more doesn't mean you are equipped to or need to. Your new rituals should help you manage stress instead of creating it. Begin with only one or two new things that can be seamlessly woven into your day and be realistic about the time your new rituals will require. Rituals don't need to be elaborate to be effective. Radical upsets only rev up your nervous system, which appreciates having a greater sense of ease into change. If you're not a morning person or you're constantly late to work, it isn't rational to think you'll be able to get up earlier to carry out a fresh thirty-minute routine *and* be on time afterward. And if your evening rituals consist of a sleepy tea, journaling, meditation, and breathing exercises, but you're working so late that committing to all of these will push back your bedtime to an unreasonable hour, it's wise to only choose those you feel are absolutely necessary or most enjoyable. Sometimes we let what we "should be doing" rule us and guilt us into being even more overextended, but the smart thing to do is to temporarily cut back.

5. LET IT BE EASEFUL

There are those that seek out the easiest route for everything and those that end up making things more difficult for themselves. A shift in mindset may be necessary if you fall in one of these extreme camps. If you're the former, you need to learn there is honor in hard work. If you're the latter, acknowledge that there are grooves in nature for a reason: The universe doesn't want you to struggle all the time. Wouldn't it be a win-win if the best solution was also the easiest one?

It may be presumptuous to say that most of us need a change because we're overbooked or overcommitted, but societal patterns—including patterns of diseases such as anxiety and depression—are hinting at this. Rather than assuming that the effectiveness of your self-care has a direct relationship to its complexity, come to terms with the idea that some of the easiest and most basic changes can be the most transformative ones.

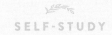

SELF-STUDY

Based on what you have learned about yourself, should your approach be to modify current rituals or to add something new? Are there foreseeable obstacles you should account for in planning a change in your routine?

Though it would seem that there is never a wrong time to incorporate actions that make you healthier, remember you're rocking the boat by modifying or altering your routine. Like an herb that has a lengthy list of both benefits and contraindications, there is very little that is purely positive if all the conditions for its success aren't met. Honing in on ideal timing can secure your success.

Be aware of logistical interruptions to rituals, such as upcoming travel. If you're trying to develop a new daily routine, but you're not going to be in your own city or home, it will be especially challenging to have any kind of consistency. At the same time, it might be an opportunity to fine-tune your travel rituals—the things you can take with you wherever you are, and ways to overcome imbalances from being someplace new.

If you've just experienced trauma or have gone through an excessive amount of change, it isn't the right time to initiate new rituals. Ayurveda always seeks to find the root cause of our afflictions, so in theory, starting the healing process closer to the time of trauma would be most effective. There is merit in allowing yourself to fully feel and process your emotions, instead of "getting over it," but there must be some transition time before you give consideration to a lifestyle change. A radical shift after being let go from a job or after the death of a loved one isn't likely to be a sound decision. Instead, sit with your thoughts. When you feel confident things have settled, and it isn't just a matter of feeling like you "should" be ready, then you can further assess if it is an appropriate time to begin.

7. CONNECT THE RITUAL TO THE VALUES IT REPRESENTS

To boost your follow-through on your rituals, it is important to steep in the feelings that you experience when you participate fully. When you have experiential evidence and embody the positive impact, there's a greater chance of your repeating the act.

A basic but significant practice for accomplishing this is writing. Keep a journal to reflect any shifts you might experience as a result of your newly incorporated rituals. (The Self-Study prompts throughout this book can be a starting-off point as you develop your own journaling practice.) That way, you have something to look back on if you are in need of motivation.

Leaving yourself ritualistic love notes is another idea. In the present moment, after you've carried out your ritual, write a couple of lines letting yourself know how what you're doing is meaningful. Leave the note in a place where you'll see it often or where you'll need it most. If waking up early and going for a walk makes you feel like you are in control of your day, write it down and leave it on your bedside table so you see it in the morning. The current you knows the future you pretty well. Use it to your advantage.

PART 4

Rituals
for
How You Feel

CHAPTER 10

How We Get Sick

The Ayurvedic Perspective on Illnesses

You can boast about having the most pristine, regular, and hygienic routine and still become sick. That's because what we experience as disease is prevented not only by eating the healthiest foods, obsessively washing our hands, and sneezing into our elbows; as we've seen, there are greater principles at play when it comes to determining our overall health status.

To be healthy, according to Ayurveda, means to be in harmony with nature and to have a state of balance of the doshas that corresponds to your unique constitution or *prakruti*. Your well-being is a reflection of your inner health; thus your mind, senses, and consciousness must be as well-functioning as your digestion and immune system.

There are three primary reasons why balance may not exist. These principles are like a warning label stuck to our modern lifestyle, explaining why the pace of life and work can feel unsuitable to our own biology. We use immune-boosting supplements and understand that managing stress is important, but we are still far from aligning ourselves with the idea that listening to nature's wisdom and our own intuition can be the preventive health measures we actually need.

1. Going against time, nature, and biological rhythm (*kalaparinama*)

The most crucial health risk factor is the disregard for the relationship between time, nature, and our biological rhythms. When we don't feel well, our first instinct is to blame bacteria or a virus, as well as those days we fell off our diets or didn't get enough exercise. Yet at the heart of even these (real) causes of disease is timing. The Sanskrit word *kala* means time, and *kalaparinama* translates to disharmony with nature, or failure to respect time with regards to the twenty-four-hour clock, the seasons, and our own internal timing. This is Ayurveda's first fundamental cause of illness, but the one that can most easily be overlooked. Eating, exercising, or sleeping at the wrong hours or failing to make changes in accordance with the seasons increases our vulnerability to illnesses that might otherwise not penetrate our system.

Western medicine refers to this as *circadian misalignment*. From our ease in accessing food and the ability to consume it any time of day or night, to constant exposure to blue light emitted from smartphones, tablets, and computers, these factors are antagonistic to our health. Science is now showing the truth Ayurveda always knew, that our maladjusted circadian rhythms are contributing to a host of illnesses, such as obesity, diabetes, heart problems, and insomnia.

2. Failure to follow your intellect (*prajnaparadha*)

When we have flawed judgment and perceptions, disregard for our past experiences, or little value for our own intuition, improper action and illness follow. For example, if you indulge in a food or behavior that you know is unhealthy, you must also know that it can have its consequences. Or similarly, if we ignore our hunger, or suppress other natural urges such as sneezing, crying, or sleeping, we will also become sick.

Though there can be mental anguish and behavioral disorders as a result of prajnaparadha, it can also cause physical harm. Substance abuse, car accidents, and even some infections can be the result of one bad decision or many. And of course, we're bound to make bad decisions or choose fun over health sometimes, but repeating this will ultimately make us sick.

3. Misuse of the senses (*asatmyendriyartha samyoga*)

Healthy senses are vital for our well-being because they are how we internalize the outer world. An external object or stimulus has to be processed by the mind before it can become an observation, thought, or perception. Without a finely tuned perception of our surroundings, we decrease our chances for survival. This was especially true when civilization was less developed and we lacked the security of shelter, electricity, and technology; then, we were alerted to danger through sight, smell, taste, sound, and touch. Today, it isn't typically a bear or a mountain lion that we need to worry about, but stress disorders.

As we sit behind screens, we no longer collect sensory experiences in real life or real time, which leads to our being under-stimulated. We lack the stimulation needed to exercise our senses the way that would make them stronger. We see picturesque landscapes, but may not experience them by smelling the mountain air, hearing birds sing, tasting salt water on our lips, or feeling the ground with our bare feet. At the same time, there is so much information and mental input coming in at one time that we are over-stimulated. We have multiple email accounts, receive

SELF-STUDY

Look beyond what you eat and how you exercise as a measure of health. In what ways do you make a conscious effort to stay connected to nature? Do you often find yourself going against your best judgment? Are you adept at using your senses and can you see their relevance to your well-being? Free of criticism, note where among the three causes of illness there may be room for improvement for you. The goal isn't to be perfect, only to strive for our best and to allow for grace when that feels impossible.

text messages and alerts on our devices at all hours, and spend the days under fluorescent lighting. It's too much for us to interpret and process. With the decreasing efficacy of our senses, the bridge between our outer and inner world diminishes.

When you witness yourself in violation of one of these three foundational causes of illness, you'll notice a trickle-down effect occurs. Offense to one almost always means there will be offense to another. You could break the rules of nature by staying up past the time your body signals you to sleep. This could lead to you eating too late at night, or in a moment of weakness cause you to eat something that you know isn't good for your health. Or maybe you decide to eat as you answer emails on your computer. As your senses are overloaded with the information from the messages you're sending, you're not in tune with the taste of the food that you are consuming and end up in digestive distress. Once your actions become patterned, it becomes harder to reconnect to your inner world.

Rituals, however, are a way to keep ourselves educated about and in tune with our internal and external realities. When we let ourselves align with nature's ways, what is best and healthiest for us will appear clearly and instinctually. As we feel better, we're more likely to make more conscious and informed decisions, to know what's best for us in any given moment, and to recognize when it's time for a change.

CHAPTER 11

Healing Rituals

Practices for Balance When You Feel Unwell

We are instinctively drawn to natural medicines, such as Ayurveda, because of the system's willingness to see things holistically instead of in parts. There's an understanding that symptoms are often related and that the entire being should be evaluated and treated. For every illness, there is a story, and healing is much more than taking a pill or a tablet to feel better, even if that pill or tablet is natural. Herbal therapies, and sometimes even pharmaceuticals, can be a necessary support on your quest to feel better. But to get better and stay better, you must consider how you got to this point in the first place and the lifestyle changes needed to turn things around.

As we learned in chapter 10, there are degrees to which imbalances and illness can be manifested. There are our smaller daily, or seasonal imbalances that come from a hiccup in our routine or diet. With a little conscious work, as quickly as these arise, they heal. Then, there are the more deeply seated illnesses that are an accumulation of unresolved issues and took more time to develop. These take more patience and time to heal.

In my practice as an Ayurvedic practitioner, I see a range of people with varying health concerns. There are those who want to learn more about Ayurveda as a way to enhance their already good health, people who are dealing with minimal symptoms, and those who have come to me as a last resort because nothing else has given them the relief that they seek. In all cases, no matter their severity, we address their daily routine and rituals. Without this as a foundation, superficial changes, including herbs and diet, won't have the same capabilities to heal, and often the source of the problem is never revealed or addressed.

The following is a list of conditions I chose based on my experiences in clinical practice. They are the most common conditions I see that are caused by or complicated by sporadic scheduling or misalignment with nature's rhythms. Patients with these conditions have had a positive response to resetting their lives with rituals, and are often surprised by how powerfully a commitment to consistency can improve how they feel. For each condition, there is an Ayurvedic explanation that uses the doshas, elements, and gunas (refer to the chart on pages 44–45). You'll find this to be a fresh perspective and a way to simplify conditions that feel complex. Even if you feel well and aren't experiencing any of these conditions, reading through them will be an educational tool; you may even notice that you have symptoms but weren't fully aware of them. This will deepen your understanding of Ayurveda and serve as a preventive source of inspiration, to help you identify potential imbalances before you become symptomatic.

Then, suggestions for morning, midday, and evening healing rituals are given for each condition. There are medicinal tonics and elixirs, breathing exercises, yoga postures (*asanas*), and journal prompts to get you going in the right direction. These can be adopted by anyone looking for additional soul-nurturing acts to incorporate into their life.

All of these healing rituals were designed with the modern world in mind, by including components of traditional Ayurveda, but keeping them easy and accessible. They are approachable as they're simplistic, and complementary without being overwhelming, and most can be completed in approximately ten minutes once you have familiarized yourself with the process. Though some of the rituals may need an additional tool or ingredient that you don't have, the idea is to aim for rituals involving things you might already have or can obtain easily and inexpensively. You'll find there are options to upgrade rituals with herbs or other tools when appropriate. More information about the benefits of these herbs or other supplements can be found in the Glossary of Herbs that starts on page 267.

You don't have to go into this full force. A few suggestions on how to begin:

1. Select only one ritual from the entire list. This should be the easiest and most appealing ritual for you. Once this feels fully integrated into your life, consider adding more. This approach is especially effective if you are perpetually feeling short on time or low on energy.

2. Choose three rituals, one each from the morning, midday, and evening. Generally, two weeks gives you enough time to become consistent and to determine if a ritual is beneficial. After the two-week period, add one more from each time of day. While anyone can begin in this manner, this is usually most successful with people that already have a steady schedule and are modifying more than they are adding.

3. Start with the complete set of rituals for only morning, midday, *or* evening. This is a great way to embrace the idea of rituals for those of you who have a time of day that is a standard period for being stressed, tired, or anxious.

Please note, what you read here is not meant to replace any care, exam, or diagnosis you receive from your healthcare or Ayurvedic practitioner. Consider it a launching point, stepping stone, or complement to the help you receive from your doctor.

Acne or Lackluster Complexion

We want to face the world with radiant skin, so whether it is because of the occasional blemish, cystic acne, or skin that lacks luster, it can be easy to lose confidence when we aren't comfortable in our skin.

Your skin is a pitta organ, and while anyone could experience a skin condition, the fiery-natured ones are the ones who will go through it most. And though there will be some involvement of pitta in all skin conditions, any of the three doshas could be at the root of the cause. For example, vata acne tends to be hard, often on the forehead, and without anything to extract. Pitta acne is red and due to the relationship to hormones, can show up around your chin and mouth. Blackheads are also related to pitta. Kaphas have incredible skin, but they aren't immune to blemishes. Theirs are typically due to excess oil and thus will look white with a whitish substance that can be extracted.

The following rituals will give your skin a boost in clarity, elasticity, and glow, no matter your dosha. Get into the groove with these different practices first, and then you can look to more dosha-related diet and lifestyle changes to help elevate your routine.

Morning Rituals

OIL CLEANSING (5 MINUTES)

It can be scary to add oil to your face if you're concerned about acne, but washing your face with a soap or face wash can be drying and disrupt the natural balance of oils. Oil will pick up dirt to be rinsed away without stripping your face of its own hydration.

You can find oil cleansers that are formulated specifically for your face, but you can just as easily use jojoba oil. This oil has a neutral smell and most closely matches your skin's sebum. Place a dime-to-nickel-size amount in your hands and gently massage it into your face. Place a warm, wet washcloth over your face and lightly press it into your skin. You can rinse the cloth and repeat if necessary; otherwise, use a towel to blot your skin dry. Unless you are particularly dry or it is a dry season, you could possibly go without any additional moisturizer after cleansing.

READING YOUR FACIAL LINES

Ayurveda uses the lines of the face as a way of diagnosing or confirming different health conditions. When there are horizontal lines across your forehead, this is from excessive worry. Two vertical lines between your eyes will appear if you have suppressed anger in your liver (on the right), or if you are holding emotions in your spleen (on the left). And deep lines that run from your nose to the outer corners of your mouth indicate poor nutrient absorption.

HIBISCUS TEA (5 MINUTES)

It can't be a coincidence that a beautiful summer flower also works in favor of a healthy complexion. Hibiscus is a cooling herb that purifies physically and spiritually and helps to clear skin and promote hair growth. In the summer, you could have this tea slightly chilled (but not cold or iced) for an extra-refreshing treat.

1 teaspoon dried hibiscus flower or hibiscus tea, or 1 tea sachet

1 cup (240 ml) hot filtered water

Optional medicinal herb boost: ½–1 teaspoon gotu kola   *recipe continues*

Place the hibiscus in a tea infuser and into your mug of hot water. Allow it to steep for at least five minutes, or longer for a stronger taste. If you are using gotu kola, you can add at the time of the hibiscus and stir thoroughly. It may not dissolve entirely and it could be strained if you prefer. If you wish, add a slice of fresh lemon or lime to complement the floral taste of the hibiscus.

Although warm or hot liquids are preferred for digestive purposes, this in no way means that they should be boiling or scalding hot at the time of consumption. Though there is variance, herbal teas or infusions generally should be steeped at boiling point, while green and black teas have a brewing temperature range between 150 and 190 degrees Fahrenheit.

Midday Rituals

LION'S BREATH (SIMHASANA) (3 MINUTES)

This breathing practice is like yoga for your facial muscles—uplifting and fun to do. As the name suggests, it mimics the breathing and facial expression of a lion, full roar. This is typically done in a kneeling position, but you could try this in another seated position, standing, or even while in another yoga pose. With your hands resting on your knees, palms down, begin to take deeper breaths. After a deep inhale, pause, full of breath. Then, open your mouth and exhale, making a big "ha" sound, while sticking out your tongue, stretching your face, and gazing toward your forehead. Your roar, or exhale, should be a steady breath that uses your abdominal muscles to force the air out of your lungs. Repeat this one or two more times. When you are finished, sit quietly with your eyes closed, feeling the energy circulate your being.

Snackers beware! Some of the things you're likely to grab to tide you over until dinnertime or to give you some fuel for your workout before dinner could be taxing your digestive system and leading to more skin problems. Most convenient foods are often processed or salty and should be reduced in your diet significantly, but one that may come as a surprise is nuts. It's easy to grab a handful of almonds or cashews and feel satiated; however, they are both heating and difficult to digest, and could easily make acne worse. Instead have fruit, which is easy to digest, or seeds, which are cooling. Both will be filling and good for your skin.

REFRESH WITH ROSE (1 MINUTE)

This ritual really proves how something small can be very powerful. Rose hydrosol is water that has been distilled from the plant, but still contains the essence and medicinal properties. In any form, rose is hydrating and cooling; and as a floral, it is a good reminder for pitta constitutions to soften their natural intensity. Rose hydrosol is a wonderful midday pick-me-up in addition to being a superb toner for your skin. Keep a bottle at your desk or in your car and make it routine to mist your face at least once in the middle of the day.

Evening Rituals

Forward bends are excellent for diffusing heat and because they take your head lower than your heart, which promotes the flow of oxygen and blood to your head and face.

A wide-leg forward bend is a friendly pose for those with restrictions in their hamstrings and lower back muscles. Planting your feet wider makes it easier to elongate your spine and bend from your hips instead of your waist. For this yoga posture, stand with your feet very far apart, about the distance between your hands when your arms are stretched out from your shoulders. Rotate your legs inward, so that your knees and toes are slightly turned in. Breathe in, bringing your arms out wide and overhead. Breathe out, sweeping your arms around in a circle and starting to hinge forward from your hips. Allow your hands to touch something connected to the ground, either the floor, a yoga block, or a chair. Inhale and lengthen your spine again, reaching the top of your head forward. As you exhale, see if you can soften further and fold a little deeper, releasing your head toward the ground. You can keep your knees bent as much as you need while you stay in the pose for five to ten breaths. Gradually come back up to standing. You can repeat one or two more times.

When your skin isn't as clear as you'd like it to be, it's easy to become hyper-focused on it when you look in the mirror. This extra stress takes away from the foundation that you are trying to build for your skin to glow. Instead, take time to journal about the beauty that exists that you may be overlooking.

Those around you look past the things you are most critical about and see your true beauty. What are the beautiful things your loved ones appreciate most about you? For your journaling prompt, take five minutes to write down the things you know others value in you. When you get stuck or distracted, refocus yourself by writing or saying, "I see the beauty that others see in me."

Adrenal Fatigue

Adrenal fatigue is a condition caused by chronic stress, something that has come to define modern Western culture. It happens when you are testing your limits by participating in more than you really have energy to sustain. You are either going so fast that you don't notice the signs of not feeling well, or you decidedly push through them. This results in a chronic stimulation of your sympathetic nervous system (fight or flight) without the balance of your parasympathetic nervous system (rest and digest). What should be a natural ebb and flow turns into an elevated baseline where your body is always prepping for survival.

Your adrenal glands do their best to regulate the production of stress hormones such as adrenaline and cortisol, but eventually even they get tired and can't keep up. You start to experience symptoms like extreme fatigue, salt cravings, anxiety, depression, and difficulty managing minorly stressful situations. It becomes more complicated when your body perceives itself to be in survival mode and uses energy for functions needed to stay alive, at the expense of otherse that aren't immediately needed, such as reproduction. In other words, if you're being chased by a bear the ability to conceive isn't a priority; energy that would otherwise be spent regulating reproductive hormones gets redirected to regulating respiration and heart rate. When you reach this point, the stress you've experienced has been accumulating for so long that your body can't recover unless a change is made.

The solution is always to slow down and choose rejuvenation over stimulation. But often the lifestyle that leads to adrenal fatigue in the first place won't allow the time for restoration. The answer then lies in the ability to give your energy a container. Those who are vulnerable to adrenal fatigue are like a garden hose turned on high without anyone holding on to it: The energy is flying all over the place, on the ground and in the air. When this happens to us physiologically and psychologically, we need to create structure and organization around our day to contain our energy and let us control where to use it.

The rituals for adrenal fatigue are specially designed to take a minimal amount of time and effort while giving your nervous system an impactful and much-needed break. Emphasis should be placed on being consistent and present, so that you can be more aware of how you feel and notice when it is time to pause before you get too overloaded.

Morning Rituals

Lemon essential oil is a known supporter of adrenal function. In general, it provides an uplifting feeling without being overstimulating. As stress can cause us to feel like we are living more in our head than in our physical body, this ritual will restore the connection as it helps to reestablish balance in your adrenal glands. Open your palms and look at your hands. Note the details, like if the shape of your palm is square or round, if your fingers are long or short, and if the lines on your palm are deep or shallow and plentiful. Be reminded of the ways your hands are a part of your day through cooking, working, playing, and helping others. Place a few drops of lemon essential oil, mixed into a teaspoon of a neutral-smelling carrier oil (such as jojoba or sweet almond oil), into your hands and rub together. Open your palms a few inches in front of your face and take in three deep breaths. Massage any excess oil onto your neck and shoulders.

Do away with your "snooze" habit, or at least be realistic about it. When your intention to get up at 6 AM is met with forty-five minutes of hitting the snooze button, you start your day feeling like you failed. The reality is, if you're hitting snooze every day, your early wake-up time isn't working out. Instead, set your alarm for the time you normally get up, which is usually the latest you can get up without being late, and you'll give yourself more uninterrupted sleep. You'll wake up feeling refreshed, and sometimes without an alarm!

Take three to five minutes to write out your daily energy budget. This is a chance to become conscious of your energy reserves, and to become well versed in the art of letting go. These prompts are designed to help you wisely budget your energy for the day. You can keep them in a journal, or write them on a piece of paper to keep in your pocket as a reminder. Creating a note on your phone can also be helpful, but avoid this step if you are easily distracted by digital devices.

I will allow space in my energy budget today to:

_____ _____.

Example: I will allow space in my energy budget today to: take a midafternoon walk outside.

Being conscious of my energy use is important because:

_____.

Example: Being conscious of my energy use is important because: my desire to give energy to others can't be fulfilled unless I have energy myself.

Midday Rituals

BE WITH NATURE (10 MINUTES)

Fancy spas and retreat centers are situated in beautiful settings for a reason. Nature feels like an escape and can be instrumental in healing. It signals us to slow down, but also reminds us that we are a small part of something much greater.

> As you are healing from adrenal fatigue, the foods you choose to nourish your body should be easy to process but also rejuvenating. Eat cooked foods and favor food that has a soupy or porridge-like consistency, like oatmeal, stews, and rice dishes. Increase root vegetables and squash, or other foods that share the qualities of the earth element (see page 14). Avoid foods that are crispy and crunchy, as their light qualities are shared with the air element, which you are trying to pacify or decrease.

For urban dwellers, finding a nearby park or grassy knoll is wonderful, but even a stroll in your concrete jungle works. Observe the plants that peek up through the cracks of the sidewalk or become aware of where the trees are in their life cycle. If you're in a climate where there is insufferable heat in the summer and cold in the winter, do what you can to bring nature indoors. Create a space in your office for plants, stones, or a fountain and when you can't make it outside to take in the fresh air, take a break to sit in your nature corner. These little efforts add up and help you feel like you're closer to your surroundings, putting your own personal matters into perspective.

ALTERNATE NOSTRIL BREATHING (NADI SHODHANA) (5 MINUTES)

Alternate nostril breathing is quite possibly the most neutral and balanced established breathing practice for the physical and energetic body. Its Sanskrit name, *nadi shodhana*, is a combination of *nadi*, meaning "energetic channel," and *shodhana*, meaning "to cleanse."

Our breathing cycles in such a way that we have a dominant nostril, which alternates periodically, every hour or so. Modern medicine suggests this is due to congestion, while yogic philosophy states that it is due to changes in our dominant energy.

There are thousands of energetic channels in the body, but two primary ones are situated on the right and left sides, each having an end point at the nose. The right, *pingala nadi*, represents the sun and is the more heating, masculine, or aggressive energy. The left, *ida nadi*, represents the moon and is the feminine, soft, compassionate energy. Alternate nostril breathing brings balance to these energies by cycling breath through the nose one nostril at a time.

To practice, sit upright with your left palm facing up on your lap. Using your right hand, place your first two fingers at the space between your eyes, also called the third eye. With your thumb, seal off the right nostril and breathe in through the left side. Take your ring finger to the left side, releasing your thumb, and breathe out through the right. Now, breathe in through the right side. Placing your thumb on the right and releasing your left, breathe out through the left. This completes one cycle. Breathe through a minimum of five cycles, then take one cycle of breath through both nostrils to close.

Evening Rituals

EVENING ENERGY REPORT (5 MINUTES)

Give yourself three to five minutes of writing time in the evening. If you found the morning prompts helpful, use the ones below to check in with your energy status for the day. This is not a time for judgment, only to be observant. If you don't feel like you followed through with your plans for energy conservation and refueling today, write a plan for tomorrow that will reset your course.

Today, I refueled myself by: _____
_____.

Example: Today, I refueled myself by: calling my best friend, painting for an hour, and taking a bath.

By refueling myself today, I was able to: _____
_____.

Example: By refueling myself today, I was able to: be more patient with my friends and family.

ADRENAL RESTORATION TONIC (10 MINUTES)

When you are low on energy, it is easy to reach for coffee or other caffeinated drinks that supply you with an artificial vigor. Instead, turn to this restorative and comforting nightcap (though you can enjoy it in the morning or evening, warm or at room temperature). The nut milk, coconut oil, and pinch of salt support your adrenal glands in a way that gives you a boost when needed or helps you to wind down.

    2 cups (480 ml) almond milk, homemade if possible (see pages 244–45)

    1 teaspoon coconut oil

    2 tablespoons cacao powder

    2 pitted dates, chopped

recipe continues

1 teaspoon ground cinnamon

Pinch of sea salt

½ teaspoon honey or molasses

Optional medicinal herb boost: ½–1 teaspoon gotu kola

1. Add the milk, oil, cacao, dates, cinnamon, and salt to a blender and blend until smooth, 1 to 2 minutes.

2. Transfer the mixture to a small pot. Bring to a boil, and then immediately remove from heat.

3. When the mixture has cooled to drinking temperature, add the honey or molasses and the gotu kola, if desired. Enjoy while sitting and reading your favorite book, journaling, or hanging out with your cat.

Avoid using white sugar and artificial sweeteners, as they tend to be overly processed or chemical-based. For adrenal fatigue or vata-predominant conditions, choose honey and molasses. Both have a slow quality (imagine being able to slow down your life to the pace of pouring honey or molasses) and generate a heating effect in the body.

Anger

Even the most open-minded and well-supported people can get angry from time to time—in fact, they may be even more susceptible to outbursts if they're constantly expected to maintain a peachy demeanor. Finding the proper outlet for expressing grumpiness is tricky, and often venting can feel like the "healthiest" solution. Still, if you feel angry, it's best to temporarily simmer in the emotion instead of dismissing it, all while being careful not to become reactive. To bury anger means that it won't be addressed appropriately and will likely build and lead to more serious issues—as is the case with most negative energy in the body and mind.

Within the Ayurvedic tradition, anger is known as a hot emotion. It physically affects our digestion, heart, skin, liver, and mind—the organs we say are governed by pitta, the fire and water elements. Because there is a lot of fire in their constitution, those who are predominantly pitta are also prone to more anger. Picture a cartoon of someone who's mad: red-faced, a head filled with pressure and steam or smoke coming out of their ears. See the connection? We use phrases like "I have to let off some steam" or "cool your jets" because anger creates heat. The reciprocal notion, that heat creates anger, is also true.

To adequately calm and defuse anger, we must defuse this heat. We can do this by minimizing food and experiences that are warm and spicy, or we can increase food and experiences that are cooler (see Table 3, page 97). It's also vital that the anger be balanced with compassion and love. You'll find the following rituals to be cool, gentle, and full of self-care. They are great for balancing anger and its counterparts of frustration, irritability, and judgment. If your primary dosha is pitta or you have a predisposition to respond to stress with anger, these rituals are a good prevention strategy.

Morning Rituals

WRITE YOUR BLESSINGS (5 MINUTES)

It seems that gratitude journaling found its way into mainstream society thanks to Oprah and the like, but in truth the practice was up for a resurgence. Gratitude is said to be one of the closest emotions to love, and when we open ourselves to being thankful for the people, places, and experiences in our lives, we get one step closer to loving ourselves fully. Take three to five minutes each morning to write at least three things for which you're grateful. Write the first things that come to mind; don't overthink it.

HEARTFELT MASSAGE (3 MINUTES)

Both receiving massage from others and massaging your own body provide benefits for so many emotional conditions, because of massage's ability to connect the emotional and the physical through touch. For anger, we try to bring everything back to the physical and emotional heart space, including massage.

For this heartfelt massage, you'll use a quarter-size drop of oil in your palm: a neutral-smelling base oil like jojoba or grapeseed, which won't create heat, is nice, or you can add a few drops of rose essential oil to the base oil to increase the heart-opening effect. Gently massage the oil across the center of your chest, using a circling motion for seven or so cycles. Stop and hold both hands over your heart, right palm to chest, left hand over right. Close your eyes.

Breathe in deeply, feeling the expansion of your chest.

Breathe out deeply, feeling the steady beat of your heart.

You are what you eat, and with lunch being the biggest meal of the day, make sure it's anger-free. Make a special attempt to prepare your lunch while in a state of joy or to eat lunch with people who make you laugh. And since anger is a hot emotion, reduce foods that also have a heating energy, such as salty, spicy, sour, fermented, or acidic foods. Instead, try food that is sweet, bitter, or astringent, like dark leafy greens, grains, beans, and lentils.

Midday Rituals

CENTER TO YOUR PULSE (3 MINUTES)

In modern medicine, your pulse is the connection to your heart. In Ayurveda, your pulse is a measurement of energy and is the pathway to your true self. It is said to carry our consciousness, as well as your own unique energy and vibration. Ayurvedic practitioners use the pulse as a tool for assessing their patients' dosha and health. This practice is very advanced and it takes years of study and experience to develop accuracy with this method. It isn't only the rate or amplitude that the practitioner is assessing—but also the quality, force, and rhythm of the pulse; if it feels like it moves like a snake, a frog, or a swan. A deep pulse gives insight into your constitution, and a superficial pulse tells of your imbalances. And adding to the complexity, each of the three fingers (that are used to read the pulse) feels for one of the three doshas, along with how your tissues and organs are functioning. Though this is only one form of physical examination, some very experienced practitioners rely solely on the pulse to determine their patients' needs.

When anger manifests physically, it can have an effect on the cardiovascular system, by increasing your blood pressure and heart rate. If you can become aware of this, you can use your pulse as a meter of your emotional state and to invoke a state of calm to ensure that these changes aren't long-lasting.

Wrap the palm of your right hand around your left wrist. Place the first three fingers of your right hand on your radial pulse, which is found below the thumb on the palm-side of your wrist. This should place your first finger closest to your thumb. Press down firmly until you feel your pulse. Then, begin to lighten the pressure until you can feel your pulse in all three fingertips. If you are having difficulty finding the space where you feel your pulse evenly through each finger, or even sensing it in all three fingers, just do your best to feel your pulse in general. Once you have it, close your eyes and hold your pulse for one minute, letting your external body be a means of accessing your internal energy. Feeling your pulse brings an awareness to your inner energy by means of your external body.

HISSING BREATH (SITKARI) (3 MINUTES)

Think of this breathing practice as "letting off steam," as it mimics the sound of heat releasing through vapor. You can practice this any time you start to feel anger arise, no special body position required. With your lips parted and teeth together, inhale slowly through your mouth, letting the air move between the spaces of your teeth and along the inside of your cheeks. This makes a hissing sound and the breath should feel cool. With your mouth closed, exhale through your nose. Repeat this a total of five times.

Evening Rituals

SUPPORTED HEART OPENING ASANA (5 MINUTES)

If you were to mimic what anger looks like in your body, what shape would you take? Do you make fists, grit your teeth, and hunker down to prepare for battle? Holding anger causes us to hold tension in our flexor muscles. These are the muscles that create fists—and the ones that protect our heart by rounding forward through our chest and torso. When these muscles are engaged, we also hold in heat. In the cooler seasons, you'll see animals curled into a ball, trying to stay warm. On a hot day, they are sprawled out to let go of heat instead of conserve it.

If anger is held in our muscles and posture, could we adjust our posture to be happier? Yes! If anger creates heat, could we release heat to release anger? Of course. Here's how:

Before you settle in for sleep, try spending three to five minutes in this supportive *asana* that allows you to stretch across your chest and heart center.

Roll a blanket lengthwise. You can also use a yoga bolster if one is handy. Sit on the floor and place the edge of your blanket or bolster just above your sacrum, the wide bone at the back of your pelvis, parallel with your spine. Lie back, making sure your head rests comfortably on the rolled blanket or bolster and that there is no compression in your lower back (the prop should be supporting that curve). Your legs can be crossed, bent, or straight in front of you on the floor—whatever you find comfortable—but be sure to reach your arms out from your chest in a T shape, level with your shoulders or higher. Let your arms be passive here, palms facing up, so that you feel a gentle stretch from palm to palm and across the center of your chest.

Breathe naturally as you feel a softening around your heart.

HEAT RELEASING, HEART OPENING TONIC (5 MINUTES)

As anger accumulates, other heat-associated conditions can start to manifest, such as acid reflux, inflammatory skin conditions, thyroid disorders, and reproductive imbalances. Bring down the heat with this infusion of the calming herb chamomile and the cooling culinary herbs mint, licorice, and fennel. This will keep you mellow, so avoid it during the day if you need to stay alert for driving or meetings. It makes a great nighttime tonic.

Note: If you have high blood pressure, omit the licorice and either replace it with anise or double the fennel. These herbs don't have the exact same effect as licorice, but all three share a cooling flavor and quality. Additionally, licorice that is deglycyrrhizinated (DGL) is said to be safer for long-term use and less likely to cause an increase in blood pressure.

½ teaspoon whole fennel seeds

½ teaspoon licorice root pieces

2 fresh mint leaves or ½ teaspoon dried mint

1 teaspoon chamomile tea or dried chamomile flowers

Optional medicinal herb boost: ½–1 teaspoon arjuna powder

2 cups (480 ml) hot (not boiling) filtered water

Lightly crush the fennel, licorice, and mint with a mortar and pestle or an herb grinder. Combine with the chamomile and the arjuna, if using, and place in a tea infuser or sachet. Place into the hot water and let steep for 5 minutes, or longer for a more concentrated tonic. Remove infuser or sachet to drink.

Anxiety

Anxiety can be described as a condition of worry, concern, or nervousness, which Ayurveda attributes to an increase in vata dosha or an accumulation of the ether and air elements. Anxiety can take on many forms and everyone experiences this condition in their own unique way. Still, the unsettled feeling, disruption, tension, and jitters that accompany the condition for many could be assigned vata's descriptive words, like light, hard, and mobile.

Because no person's condition stems from a single cause, the Ayurvedic approach asks you to review your personal circumstances and to look for the influx of ether and air properties in your life. Trauma, surgery, loss of a job, change of career, a new home, a sporadic schedule, or a diet laden with raw food, dry food, cold food, or carbonated drinks can all contribute to such a state.

Practices that provide grounding, structure, and comfort will lead you to your equilibrium. These rituals are meant for situational feelings of anxiety or the cases that arise with unexpected situations or rough patches, like when you're interviewing for a job or meeting your significant other's parents. If you have a propensity for anxiety, incorporating these rituals will help you reduce and manage future cases. And while any degree of anxiety can warrant a trip to your therapist or counselor, always seek out professional intervention for conditions that are longer-lasting or more severe.

Morning Rituals

ENERGETICALLY CLEAR YOUR SPACE (3 MINUTES)

Nervous energy is palpable, whether you've been in its presence or you've been the one emitting it. After you've removed and organized any physical clutter, it's time to energetically clear your space. Historically, energetic clearing has been used in different cultures with the help of plants, such as sage or palo santo. These plants are used in ceremonies at marked times of new beginnings, or through a practice called "smudging," but they can also be used daily.

Palo santo, also called holy wood, has a very grounding, earthy scent. It's said to move out negative energy and to bring in the positive. Use palo santo by lighting it—using an unscented candle works best—and then letting the flame go out. Waive it around, so that the smoke surrounds the area you'd like to clear and surrounds your body. It doesn't burn for too long once lit, so it is perfect for small spaces or for clearing the energy around your altar or meditation nook before you meditate.

Sage is good for clearing all energy, not necessarily only the bad. You can think of it as refreshing or resetting energy, which can be useful if you are moving into a new home, setting intentions for a new cycle—such as a new moon or new season—or embarking on a new adventure. Light the bunch of sage and either hold its end or place it into a fireproof bowl. Move it around the room in a clockwise rotation, going up and down along walls and getting to areas that could be energetically stagnant, like behind doors or in corners. Essentially what you are doing is creating a "smoke bath" by letting the smoke cleanse the space. Unless you put it out, it will continue to burn once it is lit, making it perfect for clearing larger spaces. Sage has a very herbaceous scent when it burns, so be mindful of when—and around whom—you use it.

If lighting sage or palo santo doesn't appeal to you, try using incense, an oil diffuser, or a candle dedicated to this purpose. Keep these things reserved for this ritual only, rather than everyday or general use. Your intention for using them goes a long way, so selecting a scent that you enjoy is enough, though you could use palo santo, sage, or frankincense, which have can more spiritual meaning.

ABHYANGA (20 MINUTES) (SEE PAGES 72–74)

Oil holds the warm, heavy, and grounding qualities that counteract the uprooted feeling of anxiety. When you apply it through self-massage, it generates a soothing effect, helping you to instantly feel calm. Abhyanga is also one of the top ways to decrease accumulated vata, of which anxiety is an expression. Although it would be ideal to complete this full ritual every morning, leaving the oil on for twenty minutes may be too long when you're already feeling hurried. As an alternative, shorten your abhyanga to ten minutes.

> When we experience anxiety, grounding and comforting qualities in our activities and food can help to balance. In this case, "comfort food" doesn't necessarily mean fried chicken, but rather warm and hearty food like oatmeal, sweet potatoes, squash, and warm drinks. Eating raw food or snacking instead of eating full meals can make anxiety worse.

Midday Rituals

TOUCH YOUR FEET TO THE EARTH (3 MINUTES)

With anxiety being a predominantly ethereal or airy condition, it's important to keep your feet on the earth. This is necessary in a symbolic way, but also in a literal way, since doing so is therapeutic.

Take a three-to-five-minute break when you repeatedly feel anxious. Trouble identifying only one time period? Choose one that is a point of transition. Find a place that is private and free of distractions. Now, take off your shoes and socks and press your feet into the ground. Close your eyes and note the sensation of your feet in contact with solid ground and what the surface feels like against your soles.

This practice is more powerful if you can connect your feet to grass, soil, or even (indoor) natural material like concrete or wood.

In conjunction with anxiety comes worry and fear about the future. Our thought patterns get drawn into the bad things that could happen, leaving us without the realization that everything is exactly as it should be. Sometimes the circumstances don't seem in your favor, but labeling them as "bad" isn't always accurate. Even those things that feel negative in the moment are building blocks, learning experiences, and part of the path that you are supposed to be on. As you sit comfortably with your eyes closed, breathe deeply, repeating "Everything is . . ." as you inhale, and ". . . exactly as it should be" on your exhale. Do this for three minutes, then return back to your normal breathing, and slowly open your eyes.

Evening Rituals

Imagine how it feels to have someone place their hand on your shoulder, or take a moment to place your own hand on the top of your head. Notice how the minimal weight evokes a settled feeling. Heaviness counters light emotions like anxiety, which theoretically could be why your body holds on to weight, despite concerted efforts to exercise, under times of busyness or stress—to anchor and prepare yourself if danger arrives.

While your normal meditation practice could serve up something similar, this special quiet time uses weight to help with the practice of rooting down. Set a timer for three to five minutes, or longer if allowed. Lie on your back on the floor, or sit fully upright. Drape a heavy blanket, bolster, or sandbag horizontally across your pelvis or thighs. Rest comfortably with your hands on your thighs over the prop, palms face down, to encourage even more sinking in.

NOURISHING NERVE TONIC (10 MINUTES)

2 cups (480 ml) dairy milk or almond milk, homemade if possible (see pages 244–45)

1 teaspoon ground nutmeg

1 teaspoon ground cinnamon

¼ teaspoon turmeric

Maple syrup

Optional medicinal herb boost: ½–1 teaspoon dashmula

Add the milk, nutmeg, cinnamon, turmeric, maple syrup to taste, and the dashmula, if using, to a small pot over medium-high heat. Whisk or stir until fully combined. Cook until the milk is fully heated through, 7 to 10 minutes. Cool to a drinking temperature before consuming.

Burnout

Burnout isn't a diagnosed condition, but the symptoms are very real. The term was first used in 1974 by psychologist Herbert Freudenberger, when he was assessing symptoms of people who were working in caregiver positions. He observed that the continued demands from others were leading to the declining physical and mental condition of the caregivers. They were suffering from chronic exhaustion, decreased interest in their work, less motivation to perform regular daily tasks, irritability, and depression.

Sound familiar? These days, burnout can happen to anyone who fills their time with more tasks than pauses and amusement. Imagine that "pastimes" were once used to pass the time, rather than to boost our resumes. Now—now, there is no time to pass!

Pitta doshas or those with more fiery disposition are usually more at risk of burnout than their other doshic counterparts. People with this constitution are often reliable and responsible leaders, and thus are often the ones that others call upon when they need help. They also have the highest expectations for themselves with the strongest desire for accomplishments. With increased responsibilities or endless efforts to achieve goals comes an increase in heat, which is why it is no coincidence we call this condition "burnout."

If your increased responsibilities lead to more self-sacrifice and a decline in your self-care, you're at risk of physical and emotional fatigue. Ultimately the answer is to decrease or delegate responsibilities, allow more time to decompress and rest, and work on rebuilding your energy. These rituals take into consideration that you already have not enough time and too many responsibilities. All new rituals and routines should start slow, but it is key for these burnout rituals so that a sudden drop in activity doesn't cause more worry and anxiety.

The low levels of energy that result from having burnout, adrenal fatigue, or any kind of depleting condition are often confused with kapha imbalances. This is because kapha's true nature is to be slow and steady, which is easy to misinterpret as having low energy. However, excess kapha becomes balanced with more rigor, rather than with the rest and restoration that is necessary to counteract depletion. See the rituals for depression (page 190) or lymphatic stagnation (page 226) for better solutions for balancing kapha.

Morning Rituals

MEDITATION FOR SELF-CONSERVATION (5 MINUTES)

The way that meditation allows us to center ourselves makes it dually calming and reenergizing. Having a morning meditation practice gives time for pause and self-reflection so that patterns which lead toward burnout can more easily be avoided throughout the day.

For this meditation, sit in an easy, upright position. Take three deep breaths by inhaling through your nose and audibly sighing through your mouth as you exhale. Repeat five more deep breaths, breathing only through your nose. If you feel the source of your burnout comes from your inclination to care for others first, repeat with each breath, "Through caring for myself, I am able to care for others." If you feel your burnout is the result of too many goals or objectives, repeat, "Through caring for myself, I can achieve anything." Then continue to breathe naturally, sitting for five minutes.

Come back to your breath each time you become aware of your mind trailing off into other thoughts.

This breathing practice is meant to invoke the energy of the moon. In both Ayurvedic and yogic philosophy, it is believed that the right side of the body represents solar energy (*pingala nadi*), which gives you willpower and strength; but when we are stuck in an abundance of responsibilities, this energy becomes excessive, much like burning the candle at both ends. The left side of the body represents the softer, more compassionate and understanding lunar energy (*ida nadi*). This energy can become imbalanced, too, causing more insecurities or withdrawal. By breathing in through one side of the nose and out the other in a cyclical way, it is said that we can bring these energies to better balance.

When looking to simply neutralize energy, the breathing is alternated (see *nadi shodhana*, pages 167–68). When trying to release anger and heat, you'll breathe in through the left side of your nose and out through the right. This special type of breathing has been shown to immediately decrease blood pressure and heart rate.

Still with me?

To practice *chandra bhedana*, sit comfortably with your spine lengthened and upright. Place your left hand in a receptive, palm-up position on your lap. Using your right hand, fold your first two fingers into your palm. Take a natural breath in and out. Then, place your thumb on the right side of your nose and breathe in through the left side. Place your ring finger on the left side of your nose, release your thumb, and slowly breathe out through the right.

Repeat this for at least seven cycles. Practicing this in the morning will allow you to start your day feeling calm and collected, which will result in less accumulated anger throughout the day.

Many who experience burnout are involved in roles where they give their time to other people. Eating your lunch solo, with an emphasis on receiving, can encourage recharging by turning energy inward. You can also focus more on the food that you are taking in, which in the case of burnout, should be grounding, easy to digest, nutrient-dense, and full of *prana* or energy. Avoid convenient foods that are processed and sugary, as they will only give you a temporary surge of energy. Have cooked veggies, such as root vegetables and steamed greens, as well as broths and white rice, and top your dishes with seeds such as flax, hemp, or chia to provide healthy fats. Add in protein with mung beans or lentils, and if you eat meat, white fish, turkey, or chicken is best.

This breathing practice is not reserved for morning, however, so if you enjoy the effects, you may incorporate this into your evening routine, too.

Midday Rituals

When you have nothing left to give, even being in the presence of other people, sounds, or things can feel like an energetic drain. Having a moment to recalibrate without any stimuli is important for your midday transition.

Create a personal retreat for yourself by drawing the shades in your room at home or at work. Turn off anything making sound: music or audio, but also fans or anything that might be creating air movement. If all else fails, you can retreat to a bathroom where you know your privacy will be respected.

Sit where you are comfortable, either in a chair or on the floor, in a relaxed but upright position. Close your eyes, letting the silence around you or the sound of your own breath recharge your prana. This pause will be like hitting the reset button, restoring your energy and stopping stress from accumulating through the day.

We can all afford to embrace more *yin*, or moon, energy in our lives, but this is especially important for those who are in *yang* roles of leadership or as caregivers. Seated hip stretches appropriately invoke yin energy, as they slow us down and anchor us to the earth. For this hip release, sit with your legs crossed, either directly on the floor or propped up on a cushion or folded blanket. Place your hands on your knees and begin to move your torso in a circle by leaning to one side, then forward and toward the middle, then to the other side. Exaggerate the movement so as to feel a gentle stretch around your outer hips, sides, and lower back. Make ten to fifteen circles, then without an abrupt stop, circle in the other direction. After going the same amount each way, reach both arms in front of you, moving toward a restful forward bend. Relax your neck and/or let your head rest on your hands, the floor, or another support like a yoga block. After several deep breaths, slowly return to upright, letting your head be the last thing to come up.

Evening Rituals

CREATIVE TIME (15 MINUTES)

Since burnout is most likely to manifest when we have too many responsibilities, too many goals, or too many people to look after, taking some creative time can settle the score. Not only does it help you turn inward instead of extending energy outward, but also creativity has a more free-flowing and feminine energy than our more rigid and masculine goals and responsibilities. You don't have to consider yourself "creative" to complete this exercise, but if you do, this will come easily. If not, start thinking along the lines of using your imagination, doing something artistic, or making something by hand—activities such as baking, knitting, drawing, playing or listening to music, dancing, painting, or pottery. Begin with fifteen minutes of creative time, but feel free to continue with more if you find it to be soothing and a good way to disconnect from your day.

It's time to replenish your energy stores with a tonic inspired by the Ayurvedic concept of *ojas*, or our health reserves and our vitality for life (page 243). Certain foods, herbs, and spices can help to rebuild ojas, such as almond milk, ghee, dates, and cardamom. This tonic is a simple way to include many of these beneficial ingredients in one drink.

1½ cups (360 ml) almond milk, homemade if possible (see pages 244–45)

½ teaspoon ghee or coconut oil

1 teaspoon vanilla bean powder or ½ teaspoon vanilla extract

¼ teaspoon ground cardamom

½ teaspoon ground cinnamon

2 dates, pitted

Pinch of sea salt

Optional medicinal herb boost: ½ teaspoon shatavari + ½ teaspoon ashwagandha

1. Add the milk, ghee or oil, vanilla, cardamom, cinnamon, dates, salt, and shatavari and ashwagandha, if using, to a blender. Blend until smooth, 1 to 2 minutes.

2. Transfer the mixture to a small pot and bring to a boil (approximately 7 minutes). Immediately remove from the heat.

3. Stir to be sure the ingredients have blended and the herbs and spices have dissolved. Let cool to drinking temperature before enjoying.

Depression

The kapha dosha, or the constitution of earth and water, is most prone to becoming depressed, but any dosha could become overwhelmed by a depressive state, given certain circumstances. Kapha has heavy, static, dull qualities, which when healthy provides a grounded energy. When this is in excess, however, it can create a heaviness in the body, a dullness in the mind, and a stagnation of both.

When depression occurs outside of traumatic circumstances, Ayurveda offers the perspective, that as a heavy emotional state, depression could be set off or worsened by an abundance of heavy foods or a sedentary lifestyle. Other times it can result from doshas being subdued. Think about what happens if you tell an artist they can't create, an athlete they can't compete, or a bookworm they can't read? Without the things that make us thrive, we can find ourselves feeling stagnant, unmotivated, and blue.

These rituals can help give you a boost when you are feeling down, but they are not meant to be a replacement for receiving care, especially with more lasting conditions. The stigma around mental health often discourages people from seeking help, but talking with a doctor, therapist, or counselor about what you are experiencing is always recommended.

Morning Rituals

SKULL SHINING BREATH (KAPALABHATI) (3 MINUTES)

Kapalabhati, or "skull shining breath," is a breathing practice that helps to clear the body of congestion and stagnation and draws energy from the base of the spine toward the head. It's a relatively rapid breath that uses a forced exhalation, which is particularly good for decreasing or pacifying kapha dosha. It's energizing and uplifting—so if you're feeling a little blue, it's a great way to start the day.

Practice this breathing exercise on an empty stomach. Start in an upright seated position. Because you don't want to have any restriction of abdominal movement, it's best to sit with your hips elevated, such as sitting cross-legged on a blanket or bolster, or in a kneeling position. Place your hands over your navel, and fully relax your abdomen (this is necessary for this breathing practice, despite our being programmed to suck in our stomachs when trying to sit or stand with proper posture). Now, place your palms down on your knees, and begin breathing in and out through your nose. When you are ready, exhale forcefully as if you were blowing your nose into a tissue, drawing your navel back toward your spine in a quick movement, giving a gentle contraction to your abdominal muscles. Then relax your abdomen, and let your inhale breath happen passively. Do this for twenty breaths. Breathe at a rapid rate, but not so quick that you can't maintain the rhythm. In time, you can increase the number of breaths to one hundred, or in other words, increase the number of cycles to five.

Skull shining breath is contraindicated if you are pregnant, due to the rapid abdominal movement required to perform it. You should also refrain from this breathing practice if you feel light-headed or dizzy, or if you have high blood pressure.

The lemon and ginger in this drink are invigorating and help to create a warming and circulating effect in the body.

Juice from ½ lemon

2 slices fresh ginger or ½ teaspoon ground ginger

2 cups (480 ml) hot (not boiling) filtered water

Optional medicinal herb boost: ½ –1 teaspoon mucuna pruriens powder

Add the lemon juice, ginger, and mucuna pruriens, if using, to the hot water. Stir and allow it to steep for five minutes, or until it is cool enough to drink. If you added mucuna, you may prefer to strain it before consuming, as often the powder does not fully dissolve.

Midday Rituals

Depression can be accompanied by sluggish digestion, so emphasize lighter food that has a shorter digestion time, and eat fresh rather than packaged food. Eat lots of fruit and vegetables and reduce your consumption of dairy and meat. Having fruit alone is a good option for breakfast, especially if you have cooked fruit (baked pears or apples with uplifting/warming spices such as cinnamon, ginger, or cardamom). For lunch and dinner, limit your meat intake and significantly reduce cheese, yogurt, ice cream, or cream-based dishes, as these will weigh you down. In the evening, eating in this light way is important because our digestion slows at night. Keep dinner small and easy to digest, such as some steamed veggies with a bowl of broth. Beans and legumes are good, but well-cooked vegetables and leafy greens and broth-based soups are best.

We're already prone to a dip in energy post-lunch, but if you're experiencing a bout of depression it may drag you down even more. Some movement, like light walking, could help you feel more alert, but scent is another, more portable option.

Aromatherapy has a two-fold benefit of providing scent and revitalizing breathwork. For this exercise, you'll use peppermint and basil essential both of which both can be used as mental stimulants. In a 4-ounce (125-ml) spray bottle, mix 15 drops of peppermint essential oil, 10 drops of basil essential oil, 2 ounces (30 ml) water, and 2 ounces (30 ml) witch hazel. Shake gently. Spray into the air when you need a mood boost.

> Inhaling aromatherapy stimulates the limbic system, or the part of our brain that controls emotion and stores memories. Thus, one of the fastest ways to bring about a change in mood is through scent. If you are pregnant, avoid this blend; use only lavender essential oil, but still check with your doctor before use.

A depressive state can cause you to slump in a posture with rounded shoulders, so this midday ritual is designed for you to feel more expansive and mobile through your upper body.

Find a steady, grounded stance with your feet slightly wider than your hips and your knees slightly bent. Bring your hands together at your heart. As you inhale, reach your arms straight out in front of your chest at shoulder height with your palms together like an arrow. Spread your arms wide apart as if you were ready to receive a giant hug. Exhale and reverse the movement, drawing your straight arms toward the midline, joining your palms and bringing your hands back in toward your heart. Find a quick, but safe, rhythm with this movement, where it takes one second to inhale and open your arms and one second to exhale and bring your hands back to your chest. Inhale to expand your ribcage and exhale with vigor. Repeat the movement for thirty seconds.

> The seat of kapha is in the chest, so movements that create an expansive movement across the chest are especially helpful for keeping kapha dosha healthy. Backbends, shoulder stretches, and twists that involve the upper back are among the yoga asanas that fit this category.

Evening Rituals

ADD TO YOUR "TA-DA" LIST (5 MINUTES)

Colorful sticky notes usually get filled with important tasks that we need neon colors to remind us of—but they rarely get filled with a list of things we're proud of. So using your brightly colored paper and pens, write down the day's "ta-das," or the things that you're happy to say that you accomplished for the day. Let this be your personal brag list, a giant pat on the back, a gentle stroke of your ego. For an uplifting surprise, put your list inside a notebook, coat pocket, or closet door where you might find them unexpectedly.

Sit and write down the things that you feel are weighing on you or keeping you stuck where you are. Then, in an easy seated position with an upright spine, let your palms face upward on your thighs. Breathe naturally and close your eyes. Imagine that you are wearing a backpack that holds all of the heavy items you just listed. Visualize yourself taking off the backpack and the relief you get from removing your heavy pack. Notice how your neck and shoulders relax and how there is more room and ability to breathe. Picture yourself opening the backpack, and start to remove the items one by one. With each thing you remove, state "I choose to release *X*." Once the pack is finally empty, breathe one big sigh of release.

Digestion and Elimination Problems

Both Ayurveda and Western medicine see linkages between emotional and mental states and how we break down, assimilate, and eliminate food. Ayurveda states that *agni*, the main digestive fire, is located within the lower stomach and small intestine. Should we have past traumas left unresolved or current anxiety, fear, or anger, this can greatly our digestion. You may have experienced this yourself, if you've ever had a nervous stomach or a knot in your abdomen. In Western medicine, we see more and more research going into the enteric nervous system, the network of nerves that surrounds the gut known as the second brain. From this research, we know that more than 90 percent of the neurotransmitter serotonin is produced here. This means that through the gut-brain connection, we can see digestive problems creating issues with our emotional and mental faculties, and vice versa.

Current discussion of digestive health deals a lot with the gut's microbiome, or the healthy bacteria in the gut that allow us to properly break down food. Though Ayurveda doesn't specifically discuss the microbiome, this concept is very much aligned with the Ayurvedic guidelines for eating as our microbiome also has a seasonal cycle. The bacteria in our gut fluctuate as our weather shifts from dry to wet, and from hot to cold. This is because microbes in the soil change with the season to foster the growth of different plants. Eating seasonal and local food can keep us synced with this cycle, so it is more likely that we will properly process what we eat and create a line of defense against seasonal illnesses.

Digestive conditions can't be lumped into one all-encompassing category. Ayurveda considers four digestive states:

1. *Sama agni*: *Sama* means "balanced," and this is our most desired, but also our rarest, digestive state. Balanced digestion translates into complete absence of bloating, gas, stomach pains, or hyperacidity, and to having one to two formed bowel movements a day. Someone who has sama agni typically is also in good overall health, with a strong immune system and a clear mind.

2. *Vishama agni*: When the digestive fire is too cold or variable in how it burns, this is a condition known as *vishama agni,* or variable digestion. Symptoms could include gas, bloating, constipation, hard stool, dry stool, or elimination that varies regularly between being normal, loose, and scanty. Variable digestion is most often a result of too much ether and air—excess vata—in both one's food and approach to life. Examples include a lot of travel, a sporadic eating schedule, frequent snacking, or consuming too few fats or too many raw foods. To resolve this, steadiness and consistency are crucial, along with consuming cooked foods that are more abundant in the sweet, sour, and salty tastes rather than bitter, spicy or astringent (see Table 3, page 97).

3. *Tikshna agni*: Your digestive fire should burn bright, but as with all things, it can become unbalanced, or too hot. Digestive issues that stem from excessive heat are considered to be in the category of *tikshna agni,* agni that is sharp, hot, and/or fast, where food moves through too quickly to provide nourishment. Bowel movements that are too soft, diarrhea, ulcers, and hyperacidity are all indicative of this state. As you can imagine, an overheated digestive tract can happen as the result of consuming too many heating foods, such as food that is spicy, sour, salty, or acidic. However, this could also occur from a fiery lifestyle, like relationships or jobs that have a lot of confrontation, having a lot of goals with an expectation to always succeed, or simply having a lot of responsibilities. Any

of these pitta fuelers could be provoking from the minute they begin, or take some time to build and fester.

4. *Manda agni*: Sluggish digestion or *manda agni* comes as a result of heavy foods or a sedentary lifestyle, or a general excess in kapha. You'll know you're experiencing this type of digestion if processing and eliminating your food seems very slow or if there is mucus in your stool. Exercise can help to get things moving, along with a lighter diet low on meat, sugar, and dairy.

Because of these variations, finding a blanket remedy for problems that originate from a host of issues is quite challenging; you may hear something advertised as being good for digestion that is not be good for *your* digestion. What works for constipation (cold) will not work for loose stools or acid reflux (hot). You may even find that some symptoms cross over into many categories. The following rituals are an attempt at providing neutral solutions that you can benefit from, no matter if you're running too hot or too cold, too fast or too slow, or simply don't know which way you're going. The aim is to achieve *sama agni*. You'll know when your digestive system has found its balance when you are eliminating a formed bowel movement one to two times per day, are free of any bloating or gas, and have a healthy appetite before you eat.

Your main digestive fire is located in the center of your abdomen. You can do a quick assessment to see if your fire is too low by placing your palm across your navel (the bare skin of your hand on the skin of your stomach). This area should feel warm to the touch, and even warmer than the temperature of your arms or legs. If it feels cool, it means your digestive fire could use a boost.

Morning Rituals

READ YOUR TONGUE (3 MINUTES)

Your tongue tells all. First thing upon waking, look at your tongue to assess any coating, cracking, or changes from how it usually appears. Then, scrape your tongue with a tongue cleaner (rather than your toothbrush) and make note of anything that is being scraped off (see pages 60–62 for a detailed explanation).

ABDOMINAL MASSAGE (3 MINUTES)

Before showering, leave time for some belly love. Use sesame oil or your favorite herbal oil to massage your abdomen in a clockwise pattern. Standing or lying down, with your hand flat on your abdomen and apply a gentle amount of pressure. Start by moving from your right pelvic bone up the right side of your abdomen. Move across your torso, under your ribs, and down the left. Continue to massage gently in this circular direction, which traces the line of your colon. This kind of external stimulation of your abdomen can help with movement on the inside, and keeping gas and bloating at bay. For additional benefit, the transdermal absorption of the oil ensures our digestive fire continues to burn steadily.

Midday Rituals

DIGESTIVE CCFT (5 MINUTES)

Cumin, coriander, and fennel may sound like a normal combination of spices, but when taken together as a tea, they become a powerful and well-known traditional remedy in Ayurvedic medicine. The reverence for this tea stems from how the herbs collectively stoke your digestive fire without producing too much heat. In a way, it's like a controlled burn, prepping you to break down what you take in. Drink a cup of cumin, corander, fennel tea (CCFT) thirty minutes before lunch.

½ teaspoon whole cumin seeds

½ teaspoon whole coriander seeds

½ teaspoon whole fennel seeds

1 cup (240 ml) hot (not boiling) filtered water

Lightly crush the cumin, coriander, and fennel seeds with a mortar and pestle so that the volatile oils can be infused into the water. Place the seeds into a tea infuser or sachet and add to the hot water. Allow to steep for five to ten minutes, drinking when it is cool enough to consume.

REST ON YOUR LEFT SIDE AFTER EATING (10 MINUTES)

It may garner some strange looks, but lying on your left side after eating can promote healthy digestion and elimination. In fact, Ayurveda recommends a short ten-minute catnap after eating.

This position helps with the entire digestive process. Lying on your left can help move food through the digestive tract into the stomach, located on the left side of the body. The organ is also then better positioned to secrete digestive enzymes it uses to break down that food. By contrast, the liver and gallbladder are located on the right side of the body, so when you lie on your left side, these organs are also better positioned to aid the movement of bile into the digestive tract so that it can begin to break down fats. The descending colon (think: moving down and out) is also on the left, so by means of gravity, resting on your left side can help waste move through your large intestine so it's ready to be ushered out the next morning.

Evening Rituals

We use tonics and tinctures to increase our digestive fire so that we can process our food, yet we often forget to enhance our emotional and mental digestion. Though our agni is strongest in the middle of the day, it can still be hindered by lingering thoughts. Before you eat your dinner, follow these steps:

1. In a place without distractions, sit quietly for a few minutes. Recall any difficult conversations or situations that have occurred over the last twenty-four hours.

2. When you think about these experiences, where do you physically feel it in your body? Does it feel like tension, pain, or another sensation?

3. For these impacted areas, create a release either by massage, movement, or stretching. For example, take your right hand to your left shoulder and rub or squeeze the area for one to three minutes, or set your feet wide apart and bend from your hips to release the backs of your legs.

4. After addressing these places, sit comfortably and still again. Take three deep breaths by inhaling through your nose and exhaling through your mouth.

As bedtime nears, use gentle movements that promote digesion, such as this yoga posture that acts as a massage for your intestines.

Lie on your back with your legs straight on the floor. Bring your right knee to your chest. You can either hold your shin or behind your right thigh. As you draw your thigh closer to you, you'll feel a slight compression of your thigh at the right side of your abdomen, or your ascending colon. Hold for thirty seconds to one minute. Release your right leg and take three deep breaths. Now, bring both knees to your chest and hold for thirty seconds to one minute. This position stimulates the transverse colon, which connects the ascending and descending sides. Release both legs straight again, and take three deep breaths into your lower abdomen. Finally, bring your left knee to your chest and hold for thirty seconds to one minute. As your left leg is drawn toward your chest, you're gently compressing the descending colon. Lay flat with both legs extended once again to conclude.

Female Hormonal Balance

Stress interferes with our physiology, and for women, it often results in a hormonal imbalance of estrogen, progesterone, and testosterone. Each will experience this in her own unique way, but symptoms can include infertility, premenstrual symptoms (PMS), uterine fibroids, ovarian cysts, irregular menstrual cycles, or symptomatic menopause with mood changes, hair loss, and hot flashes. It would be best to address each of these individually (and under the care of a healthcare practitioner), yet because the source of many of these issues is stress, there are general approaches we can use to foster a healing environment for hormonal imbalances that women experience.

> Menstrual cycles should not be symptomatic! We have come to accept PMS as being a normal thing that every woman experiences, but that isn't—and doesn't have to be—true. You can begin to work with your symptoms by identifying when they occur, pacifying the dosha at play. Symptoms during menstruation often indicate vata imbalance, occuring between menstruation to ovulation is kapha, and from the time of ovulation to menstruation is pitta. Tackling this issue on your own can be difficult, so be sure to enlist the help of your Ayurvedic practitioner.

Though the line between gender roles is beginning to blur, women still have to work harder for recognition and promotion compared to their male counterparts, often while still playing the role as the family caregiver, organizer, and manager. Determined and eager, women are the heroines to many, but this leaves them little time for exercise, a healthy diet, and self-care.

Hormones are governed by pitta or the dosha made of fire and water. The period from puberty to menopause is the pitta stage of life, and thus the time when most hormonal imbalances occur. When you couple this with a woman who is pitta predominant and working in a masculine-leaning career or environment, the effects of the imbalance become amplified.

Because the vata stage is the period of life from menopause onward, menopause symptoms can be greatly decreased by pacifying both the pitta dosha (which governs female hormones) *and* vata. In fact, those who enter menopause with accumulated vata will experience more symptoms during this transition. During menopause, it's helpful to keep a regular schedule; choose gentle exercise like walking or yoga; use oil externally; and consume healthy fats by eating more nuts, seeds, and avocados.

Morning Rituals

YIN-YANG MEDITATION (5 MINUTES)

Yin and yang are opposing energies and one is unable to exist without the other. Yin represents feminine, lunar, or cooling energy, whereas yang is masculine, solar, or heating energy. We invoke and express yin energy when we practice compassion, move slowly and freely, speak from the heart, and make decisions based on intuition. Yang is emphasized when we exercise our willpower, work hard to achieve goals, engage in competition, and work through problems with logic. In the body, the left side represents yin energy and the right represents yang. This meditation is about keeping these energies in check, so that it can become evident when we've been pushing too hard to manage the responsibilities of home, work, and personal life without time to retreat for the self-nurturing acts we need.

Begin seated with your back upright. Turn your palms face up, with your elbows bent and hands at midchest height. Inhale and feel the yang energy of the muscles supporting you through your back and abdomen; exhale and feel the softness of the yin energy around your neck, shoulders, and hips. Now, think of the aspects of your current life that represent yin energy and imagine holding them in your left hand. How heavy or light does this feel? Think of the activities in your life that represent yang energy and hold them in your right hand. How does the weight feel in your right hand? Compare your two hands—is one more heavily weighted? Visualize the ways you can embrace these energies and allow them to be more equally represented in your life. Release your palms until they're face down on your thighs. Take three deep breaths.

BOUND ANGLE POSE (BADDHA KONASANA)
(3 MINUTES)

Also called cobbler's pose or butterfly stretch, bound angle pose is a seated stretch that releases hip muscles and tension across the pelvic floor.

Sit on the floor at the edge of a thick, folded blanket. Place the soles of your feet together, releasing your knees to the sides. Press your fingertips into the ground behind you to help elongate your spine and tip your pelvis forward until it is upright. You'll begin to feel a stretch across your inner hips and thighs. If you don't feel much at all, you can continue to press down into your hands to keep moving your upper body forward, bearing in mind that the movement should be from your hips tilting forward rather than rounding your back. With each deep inhalation, lengthen your spine. With each exhalation, soften around your hips and heavy your legs. Stay where there is a moderate, but not too intense, stretch for one to two minutes.

Midday Rituals

BALANCED BREATHING (SAMA VRITTI) (3 MINUTES)

As we stay conscious of the concept of balance in the doshas and yin and yang energies, balanced breathing is an exceptional way of keeping an equilibrium in both body and mind.

For this exercise, start with a comfortable upright seat. Start with a clearing breath by breathing in through your nose and out through your mouth. With your next inhalation, breathe in through your nose to a count of four and hold your retention for a count of four. Exhale steadily through your nose using the same four count, and hold, empty of breath, for a count of four. This completes one cycle.

This breathing exercise is recommended for the middle of the day so that it can act as a reset. Though it would be best to be in a dedicated space, or to sit on the floor with a meditation cushion or a blanket, the priority is to do this daily with consistency. Thus, you may find yourself pushing back from your desk and practicing this in your office chair, or sitting in your car with the radio off (not while driving, of course!). No matter the setting, stay present and mindful as you breathe, so that this can feel like the self-nurturing ritual that it is instead of another item on your agenda.

Retaining your breath or pausing while empty of breath can be considered an intermediate to advanced breathing practice. For some, it can cause strain, or even anxiousness or panic. If breathwork is new to you, wait to advance to this in the breathing exercises you choose.

GODDESS TONIC (3 MINUTES)

This tonic uses pomegranate as the main ingredient, which is a fruit that is beneficial to both men and women. It has a sour flavor that would typically be aggravating to pitta dosha, but this fruit is an exception and can be balancing to all doshas. It is nourishing to the heart and digestion, and is considered to be an aphrodisiac. Pomegranate is a symbol of fertility and it helps to balance estrogen levels, and is especially good for controlling the heat during menopause. The aloe vera and lemon or lime will also aid digestion, making this good to sip in the afternoon or after lunch.

1 cup (240 ml) pomegranate juice

½ cup (120 ml) room-temperature filtered water

2 tablespoons aloe vera juice

Squeeze of lemon or lime juice

Optional medicinal herb boost: ½–1 teaspoon shatavari

Add the pomegranate juice, water, and aloe vera juice to a large bowl. Stir briskly until well combined. Add a squeeze of either juice and the shatavari,

recipe continues

if using—but note that it may not fully dissolve. You can also try steeping the shatavari in the ½ cup (120 ml) hot water for 3 minutes, then straining the liquid and adding it to the pomegranate and aloe juices. Drink when at room temperature.

Evening Rituals

TAP INTO AJNA MARMA (5 MINUTES)

In chapter 6 we discussed marma points: vital areas of the body that correspond to different organs or conditions, which can be used to promote healing. For this ritual, we'll be drawing our awareness to *ajna marma*, which is located at the forehead midline, just slightly above eyebrow level, or at the space referred to as the third eye. Ajna marma is also called *sthapani*, and both names have similar meanings. *Ajna* means "order" and *sthapani* means "steadiness in the mind." While this implies balance, we use it to address female hormonal imbalance in particular because it is at the level of the pituitary gland. The pituitary gland is the master gland that releases the hormones that control all other glands. It is also a marma point that is used to relieve stress.

For this ritual, you can be either seated in your meditative posture, or reclined on your back. Be comfortable, but not so comfy that you could fall asleep. Using your left thumb, apply a gentle amount of pressure to anja marma. Continue this for five to seven breaths. Then, slowly make five circles in a clockwise direction, followed by five circles moving counterclockwise. As you release your hand from the point, let your arms rest comfortably and continue to keep your focus and attention on this point for three minutes.

Wash your worries away with an evening soak. Draw a bath or soak your feet. Let this be the time of night that is about nothing but rest and relaxation.

No matter which soak you choose, you'll use warm water, Epsom salt, cardamom essential oil, spearmint essential oil, and lavender essential oil. These oils create a calming, cooling, and grounding *tridoshic* (beneficial for all three doshas) aromatherapy blend. Soak for ten to twenty minutes, and afterward, be restful.

To warm bath water, add:	For a foot soak, add:
1 cup (150 g) Epsom salts	¼ cup (40 g) Epsom salts
5 drops cardamom essential oil	2 drops cardamom essential oil
8 drops spearmint essential oil	4 drops spearmint essential oil
10 drops lavender essential oil	5 drops lavender essential oil

Inflammatory Conditions

Every condition that falls into the inflammatory category involves an accumulation of heat, so in Ayurveda they are classified as a pitta imbalance. Inflammation can involve redness, tenderness, and a burning sensation, but does not necessarily have swelling. While fluid accumulation may accompany this process, inflammation and swelling are not one and the same.

Although it may seem logical to balance heat with cold, using ice for inflammation is not advised as it causes constriction and contraction that can close the very channels that need to be open to heal. Instead, gradually cooling with foods and calming practices are prioritized. We've seen this before, when we discussed anger, another heat-based and heat-producing condition (see pages 170–71). If you are prone to anger, you may likely be prone to inflammatory conditions, too, yet it is possible to experience one without the other.

Signs, symptoms, and diagnoses that Ayurveda treats as inflammatory or having too much heat include, but are not limited to, rashes, acne, sunburns, psoriasis, ulcers, anger, and anything ending in "-itis," a suffix that means inflammation. The rituals that follow are all-encompassing, though you may consider something more specific to the tissue that is inflamed.

Morning Rituals

"CHOOSE YOUR CHILL" DAILY AFFIRMATION
(5 MINUTES)

Mantras or affirmations are a way to refocus and align your energy. When you are experiencing an inflammatory condition, using a mantra to imply and invoke "chill" can keep you from overheating. Create a daily affirmation with words like *cool*, *calm*, *collected*, and *peaceful*, or statements like, "I am receptive to *X*," or "My mind is open to *X*."

In most situations, our technological devices can bring us more stress than calm, but here, they could come to your aid. You can either set an alarm (with a calming tone) to go off two to three times throughout the day to remind you of your affirmation. There are also apps that allow you to set reminders to pop up on your screen. Plug in your affirmation as a reminder and it will catch your attention when you most need it. If you don't want to use electronic alarms, write your affirmation down on paper and put it in your pocket.

COOLING ELIXIR (3 MINUTES)

This remedy to your inflammatory conditions includes one of the most cooling and hydrating liquids you can consume: coconut water. It's no coincidence that coconuts are grown in tropical places, as they help to keep you cool in the warm climate. While I was visiting Kerala, India, I was able to order coconut water at a restaurant and the server would bring out a fresh young coconut, cracked open with a straw stuck inside. You should be able to find young coconuts in a grocery store or market if you want to get the water straight from the source, but for the sake of ease, you can easily pick up coconut water that comes in a can or box (preferably avoiding plastic, as it is healthier, and safer for our environment).

1 sprig of mint

2 cups (480 ml) coconut water

Juice of ½ lime

Optional medicinal herb boost: ½ teaspoon guduchi

First, lightly crush the mint with a mortar and pestle. Place it in the bottom of your cup. Pour in the coconut water and stir in the lime juice. If you choose to add guduchi, you can add it directly to this mixture, or steep it first for three to five minutes in ¼ cup (60 ml) hot water. Then, strain and add to your cup. Drink when at room temperature.

Midday Rituals

According to Ayurveda, the external temperature of food has nothing to do with whether it is "cooling" or "heating." Instead, you want to reduce what creates a heating *effect* in the body and increase what has the ability to cool. In general, food that is spicy, salty, sour, acidic, or fermented will kick up the heat, but bitter, sweet, and astringent food can mellow things out. Learn more about the foods with heating and cooling energies in Table 3 on page 97.

COOLING BREATHING (SHITALI) (3 MINUTES)

Breath can be warming or cooling depending on the way you shape your mouth. Think about what you do to cool your food by blowing on it. Now picture your mouth when you try to warm your hands in winter, or fog up a window in the cold. *Shitali* breathing uses this concept. When you feel hot externally—or as though your digestion, thoughts, or emotions are festering internally—shitali will chill you out.

If you can roll your tongue, do so and breathe in through your mouth as if you were slurping your breath up through your tongue like a straw. Exhale through your nose, with a closed mouth and relaxed lips. If you can't curl your tongue, you'll simply shape your lips in a small circle, also like you were drinking through a straw, and inhale. Again, breathe out through your nose. Repeat this breath seven times, or until you feel you've regained your calm.

Use a refreshing hydrosol mist that uses the cooling power of plants to prevent heat accumulation—it is the perfect midday spritz for your face, arms and neck.

Choose your favorite scent among the most cooling plants: lavender, rose, cucumber, or chamomile. Carry this with you and use it throughout the day as a way to keep your cool, especially on the days that are most stressful.

Evening Rituals

Twists are among the most common yoga postures used to pacify pitta. This is because they are focused on the seat of pitta at the small intestine and lower part of the stomach. The wringing-out action of the twist helps to release excess heat, especially when done in the passive form of a restorative twist.

You'll need a yoga bolster or a few blankets for this ritual. If you're using blankets instead of a bolster, you'll fold them into long rectangles to support your whole torso, neck, and head. Stack enough so that the height is around six inches (15 cm).

Sit on the floor with your right hip nestled at the narrow edge of the bolster with your legs bent to the left. Turn to face the bolster, placing one hand on each side. Lengthen your spine on an inhale, and as you exhale, you'll begin to lay the front of your body across the bolster, creating a gentle twist. You can complete the twist by turning your head to the right, but if this feels stressful on your neck, keep your head turned left. Let your arms rest comfortably by your sides. Stay in this twist for three minutes. When you are ready to come out of the twist, move slowly and let your head be the last thing to come up. Repeat on the other side, with your left hip at the end of the bolster and your legs bent to the right.

JOURNAL FOR PEACE (3 MINUTES)

Emotions aren't exempt from the list of things that can create a heating or cooling response in the body. The goal is not to stop experiencing these emotions, but to understand that each needs to be processed in its own unique way. As a part of your healing from inflammation, this journal prompt focuses on the cooling emotion of peace.

Sit in a comfortable and quiet place. Take a moment to think of someone who gave you joy in your day. Write, "I am at peace with X, who brought me joy today with X." Think of someone or something who brings you challenges. Write, "I am at peace with X, despite my challenges with him/her." Finally, write, "I am at peace with myself."

Insomnia

We've come to think that it is OK to struggle to fall asleep, wake during the night, or have the occasional night of insomnia. While this may be common, trouble sleeping isn't normal. An uninterrupted night of sleep is essential for our body and brain to restore and repair, and even waking once in the night should be addressed if it is happening once or more weekly, whether or not you can readily fall back asleep.

Difficulty sleeping always involves an aggravation of vata dosha—it's an irregularity or variability with the mobile quality of air. Yet, there are still different reasons for lack of sleep that may align with another dosha. Vata is to blame when you wake up feeling cold, get up to use the bathroom, wake up with worry or racing thoughts, or wake during the vata time, between 2 and 6 AM. Pitta is responsible if the difficulty sleeping occurs between 10 PM and 2 AM, if you wake up hot, or if you wake up with a focused thought, goal, or objective on your mind. Kapha will typically cause excessive rather than interrupted sleep, but in the case of kapha-related depression, it's the excess water and earth that can keep you from a full night of rest.

The rituals listed here are centered around vata-based insomnia, but are also general enough to be practiced by any dosha or for any dosha imbalance. Sleep is one of the most researched topics within circadian medicine, so in these rituals you'll also find a large emphasis on staying linked to nature.

Morning Rituals

WAKE AND WALK WITH THE SUN (10 MINUTES)

Sleep is one of the biggest functions of our physiology related to circadian cycles. This means that our wake times can make or break us when it comes to our internal clock staying properly wound. Our body resets our circadian clock by the light cycle of the sun. Set your alarm to wake you within thirty minutes of the sunrise. The more consistent you can be with this, the more natural it will feel to fall asleep at a decent time (by 10 PM, or earlier in the winter), which works in your favor to keep you asleep the entire night. Since the sunrise changes with the season, your wake time should also adjust somewhat. Start your day earlier in the summer, and later in the winter. This will naturally allow you a more seasonally appropriate amount of sleep.

Unless it will cause a privacy issue, or a feeling of anxiety and vulnerability, sleep with your shades or blinds open. Allowing daylight to come in will help you to adjust to the sun's seasonal changes by naturally signaling you to wake. When keeping your shades open isn't possible, look into getting a sunrise alarm clock that wakes you with a light that mimics daylight and gradually increases in brightness.

Once you're waking with the sun, you'll want to get out in it. No matter the climate, getting outside and having exposure to daylight resets our melatonin cycles. Additionally, as you recall from chapter 3, the morning is a good time for exercise, playing into our natural elevation in energy.

ENERGIZING MORNING TEA (5 MINUTES)

It may be tough to get going in the morning if you didn't get a full night of rest. Rather than reaching for a caffeinated or sugary drink to move the process along, try this energizing tonic. This caffeine-free tea gives you an alert and light feeling that, unlike with caffeine, the body can sustain.

> 1 teaspoon loose rooibos (red bush) tea
>
> ½ teaspoon ground cinnamon
>
> 1 teaspoon vanilla bean powder, or ½ teaspoon vanilla extract
>
> Optional medicinal herb boost: ¼–½ teaspoon shatavari + ¼–½ teaspoon ashwagandha

2 cups (480 ml) hot (not boiling) filtered water

Honey (optional)

Add the tea, cinnamon, vanilla, and shatavari and ashwagandha, if using, to the water, and allow it to steep for five minutes. Strain, add honey, if desired, and drink to energize.

Midday Ritual

AWAKEN YOUR SPINE (5 MINUTES)

This midday ritual is for the time of day that you are most tempted to reach for a sugary snack or caffeinated drink. While these stimulants can give you a boost of energy when you need it most, they are also likely to disrupt your sleep cycle at night. Spinal movements can be just as revitalizing without the negative effects.

These awakening movements can be done seated or standing. When doing them standing, bend at your hips to place your hands on your knees. If you are seated, simply place your hands on your knees. To begin, round or curl your spine forward as you exhale. Then reverse, and create an arch or backbending movement with your inhalation. Alternate between these positions five times as you breath continuously, taking time to move your spine evenly. Next, create a "C" shape by laterally bending from side to side, moving your shoulder to your hip. Repeat this to each side five times, exhaling as you bend, and inhaling as you straighten to the center. Finally, you'll finish with five circular movements in each direction, moving your torso forward, to the side, back, and around to the other side, undulating your spine as you go along.

This is a traditional breathing practice that creates the buzzing sound of a bee. It's used to alleviate tension and reduce anxiety, but it also elicits a state of joy. Since it isn't common for adults to go around making noises in public (and, quite frankly, that's what makes this breathing practice so fun), this may be something you want to practice at home or with a closed office door. And because you're using this breath in part to stay alert, you can choose to do this with your eyes open rather than closed if you like. Sitting in your chair or on the floor, breathe several normally paced breaths in and out through your nose. Then after a deep and slow inhalation, breathe out while creating a steady high-pitched "eeee" or humming sound with your mouth closed and jaw relaxed. Repeat this for a total of three cycles.

Evening Rituals

These rituals exclude an evening drink, which could seem counterintuitive when so many natural sleep aids could be added to a nighttime tonic. The reason for this omission is that drinking too close to bedtime could cause you to wake up during the night to use the bathroom. If you'd like to have something to make you sleepy, have tea or a milky drink with herbs like valerian, passionflower, or skullcap, or spices like nutmeg, saffron, cardamom, or vanilla. Drink no more than one cup, and no later than one hour before bed.

So often it is our mind that wakes our body. A mental download before bed can prove irreplaceable for this reason, and journaling is exactly the right tool for it. To be perfectly honest, I was never one who liked journaling; it took journals that contained writing prompts for me to get hooked. When I didn't know what to write about, a question or inspirational quote would always help. If this sounds like you, search for something similar—a gratitude or happiness journal— with prompts, merely to get you in the habit of writing something before bed.

If you're totally open to the idea of writing, consider two approaches. If you wake up at night or have difficulty falling asleep because your mind is overactive and flitting from one thought to the next, journal with a recap of your day, the emotions you felt, and how you'd like tomorrow to be. If you wake with a problem-solving or hyperfocused mind, write down your to-do list before you go to bed. Circle your top three priorities. Be sure to take a few deep breaths when doing so and remind yourself that you're making a conscious decision to sleep now, so that you can have the brain power and energy to deal with those priorities with your full attention tomorrow.

SO HUM MEDITATION (5 MINUTES)

The repetition of words can help to focus our thoughts and center our mind, similar to counting sheep. Carrying much more potency than sheep, however, is the mantra *so hum*, which means "I am that" (*so* = "I am," *hum* = "that"). This meditation is meant to bring us into a state of being and to release us from our thinking mind.

Find a meditative seat with your palms placed upward on your lap. To avoid drifting off to sleep while in this settled state, it's best to sit on the floor or in your designated sacred space. Set a timer for five to ten minutes. Draw your attention to your breath and begin to deepen it, noting how your breath sounds like the phrase *so hum*—the aspirant sound of "so" as you inhale, the vibratory sound of "hum" as you exhale. With your next breath, say to yourself "so" as you breathe in, and "hum" as you breathe out. Continue this until you hear your timer. Move slowly from your seat, to settle into bed.

> If you shower or take a bath in the evening and notoriously have trouble sleeping, try bathing in the morning instead. While they are cleansing and refreshing, showers can be too stimulating for the evening, and though baths are relaxing, sometimes the warm water increases circulation, which can wake us up. If it's essential for you to cleanse at the end of your day, try using a washcloth instead, or reference the information on page 88–89.

Joint Pain

There are so many reasons why we could feel aches and pains in our joints. But whether they come from trauma or overuse or something else, Ayurveda considers all of them related to an increase in the mobile air element or vata dosha, which governs our joints and all movement in the body. Though you could have a pitta inflammation or kapha swelling in your joints, all joint conditions have vata involved primarily. This means that if there is more air element in your constitution, you could have a predisposition to joint pain; or if you experience frequent vata imbalances, you are also at a greater risk for joint problems.

The health of a joint is dependent upon many things, including having the proper support from muscles and connective tissues, the right kind and amount of motion to provide circulation of nutrients, and adequate cushioning and lubrication for protection. You'll find the rituals for healthy, pain-free joints support all of these components.

Morning Rituals

OIL YOUR JOINTS BEFORE SHOWERING (5 MINUTES)

You will be surprised at how oiling your joints externally feels like you've lubricated the surfaces on the inside. When you apply the oil, you're helping to facilitate circulation, which decreases swelling, increases blood flow, and brings nutrition to the joint. As the oil is absorbed through your skin, it keeps the muscles and soft tissue supple by directly feeding into the tissue.

When carrying out this ritual, you can use the oil that you use for your *abhyanga* (see pages 72–74), as you'll see a benefit from any oil, but there are certain ones that are superior for joints. Mahanarayan is the most traditional oil used for muscles and joints. The base oil is sesame and it is infused with herbs to help relieve pain and rejuvenate tissue. If this isn't available to you and you'd like to use an herbal oil, look for something that contains turmeric, ginger, licorice, clove, or boswellia.

You can choose to oil only your achy joints, the ones that see the most strain and repetitive movement, or all of them. Start by heating a ¼ to ½ cup (60 to 120 ml) oil, warming it either in a pot on the stove, in an oil warmer, or in a glass bottle under hot water. Place a dime-size amount in your hand and distribute it over a joint. With both hands and a gentle amount of pressure, move in a circular motion in both directions, paying extra attention to any areas where the connective tissue or muscles feel dense. Leave the oil on for a minimum of five minutes, but up to twenty minutes, before taking a warm shower and rinsing (not washing or scrubbing) the excess oil away.

TURMERIC GINGER TONIC (5 MINUTES)

Ginger and turmeric are two herbs that you can reach for to help with a multitude of conditions. In this case, they work synergistically to soothe your joints by promoting microcirculation around the joints and reducing inflammation. Fresh ginger works best for this because it is less heating and has more unctuous properties, whereas dried ginger powder is light, dry, and heating and could aggravate vata instead of pacifying it. Lastly, since this drink has an anti-inflammatory and pain-relieving effect, you may choose to have it in the evening. I have recommended it in the morning to act as a sort of warm-up before embarking on physical activity for the day.

1 inch (2.5 cm) ginger, peeled and chopped

1 teaspoon ground turmeric

2 cups (480 ml) hot (not boiling) filtered water

Optional medicinal herb boost: ½–1 teaspoon boswellia

Add the ginger and turmeric to the water, along with the boswellia, if using. Allow it to steep for five minutes. Stir or whisk to combine the ingredients and to break up any of the particles that may not have fully dissolved. Allow it to cool to drinking temperature. Strain the liquid before drinking.

Midday Rituals

JOINT FREEING MOVEMENTS (5 MINUTES)

This sequence of movements addresses all of the joints in your body. Doing this midday will reset your musculoskeletal system after prolonged sitting, standing, or repetitive movement .

You'll start with your feet and move upward, doing each designated movement five times in each direction.

1. Begin by shifting your weight onto your right foot; place the ball of your left foot on the ground. Move your left foot in a circle, shifting the weight from the ball of your foot to your toes to feel a stretch around your entire foot. Repeat this on the right side.

2. Place your feet and knees together, then bend at your knees and hips to place your hands on your thighs just above your knees. Trace circles with your knees, five times in each direction.

3. Stand up and separate your feet to hip width, hands on your hips. Trace a circle with your hips and pelvis. Make big movements, five times in each direction.

4. Move your hands to your shoulders with your elbows bent, and your feet still hip distance apart. Start to twist your spine, turning right and left, letting your elbows help lead in each direction.

5. With your hands still at your shoulders, draw big circles with your elbows, five times in each direction.

6. Release your hands from your shoulders and interlace your fingers in front of your body. Keeping your forearms close to touching, circle your hands to roll out your wrists.

7. Let your arms relax at your sides. Take a deep breath in, and on your exhalation, let your head lower toward your right shoulder. Do this without force. Inhale and bring your head back to the center, and as you exhale, lower your head to the left. Inhale to bring your head back to center. Finish the entire series by taking one deep breath.

ALTERNATE NOSTRIL BREATHING (NADI SHODHANA) (5 MINUTES) (SEE PAGES 167–69)

Intentional breathing practices can reduce pain. Not only does slowing your breath ease the effects of the sympathetic nervous system, but also it can temporarily redirect your attention from your pain. Because alternate nostril breathing is neutral in thermal effect—it isn't so heating that it will exacerbate inflammation, but it is still warm enough to encourage circulation—it makes for an ideal practice when you are experiencing joint pain.

Evening Rituals

HEAT PACKS (10 MINUTES)

Eastern medicine never adopted the now popular routine of using ice on painful muscles or joints, even after the technology for freezing was introduced to India. It's thought to be counterproductive as the cold causes a constriction of the blood vessels, preventing proper movement of lymph and blood and keeping healing nutrients from reaching the area. This is even true of inflammatory joint conditions, so long as they are not an acute injury.

Heat helps increase micro-circulation around the joint, which is essential for healing. It softens tissue, making movement at the joint easier; warm muscles stretch better and allow for increase range of motion. Moist heat is better than dry heat, as it reaches the level of the tissue you want to treat instead of warming you superficially. There are specific heating pads that provide moist heat, but you can also use a wet cloth or towel, or use oil on your skin for moisture prior to heating. Place a heating pad over the areas of your body where you feel the most pain. Leave the heat on each affected area for ten to twenty minutes.

Dealing with physical pain can be exhausting on all accounts, making us impatient with the amount of time all healing requires. In such moments, it is easier to convince yourself that you are falling apart than to realize that you are well and whole. So when you feel like you're doing all you can physically, you can nurture that process by also taking care of yourself emotionally and mentally.

Give yourself five to ten minutes before bed to reflect on how you can be present with your healing process. How can patience serve you in healing? Are you allowing yourself to be content and at peace with both your body's capabilities and its limitations? Can the idea of healing taking time actually make you more comfortable with how you feel currently, knowing that there is potential to feel better? Seek ways to be content with the way you feel now and with the fact that your body has the capability and capacity for healing. With each deep breath, repeat to yourself, "I am well. I am whole." When you are done, close your eyes, place your hands over the area of pain, and take three deep breaths. If the site isn't within arm's reach, imagine the hands of a loved one doing the same.

Lymphatic Stagnation

The lymphatic system is a part of the largest circulatory system in the body, as it works with our cardiovascular system. It's essential to our immune system, as it carries lymph, which contains white blood cells that fight infection but it has one of the largest roles in removing waste. Ayurveda has recognized lymph and the lymphatic system as important for thousands of years. In a series of seven tissues, lymph (along with plasma) is considered to be the first tissue, or *dhatu,* to form (see Table 5). This is of importance because tissues form sequentially, meaning the health of the second is reliant on the proper formation of the first, and so on. In other words, if this primary system isn't functioning, everything that comes after it—red blood cells, muscles, fat, bone, bone marrow, and reproductive organs—won't be able to do their jobs.

Table 5. Seven Tissues

TISSUE	SECONDARY TISSUE	WASTE MATERIAL
Plasma and lymph	Epidermis, breast milk, menstrual fluid	Mucus
Red blood cells	Blood vessels, small tendons	Acidic secretions, bile
Muscle	Ligaments, dermis, subcutaneous fat	Ear wax, nasal secretions, navel secretions, tartar
Fat	Tendons, omentum	Sweat
Bone	Teeth, cartilage	Nails
Bone marrow	Sclerotic fluid	Tears
Reproductive tissue	Ojas	Smegma

Lymph can become stagnant if we aren't exercising enough or if we're exposed to too many things that our body can't or shouldn't have to process, including processed foods, plastic that has leached into food, or pollution in the air. This stagnation is unhealthy because it prevents the proper removal of waste and/or proper immune function. Symptoms that arise from poor lymphatic flow most typically align with kapha imbalances, and can include fatigue, brain fog, and fluid retention or swelling. These rituals address the idea of lymph congestion, but could also be used for any general feeling of sluggishness.

Morning Rituals

LIBERATING LIFE'S STAGNATION (5 MINUTES)

Physical stagnation can manifest as emotional issues, and the emotional can manifest as physical. Round and round this story goes. Are there areas of your life where you are feeling stagnant—professionally or personally, in your creative world or your relationships? Use this journal prompt to become aware of mental and emotional stagnation and begin the journey of liberation.

Sit quietly for a few minutes to help settle your mind. Think of the challenges in your life that are on repeat, or the roadblocks that you continue to come up against. Now, visualize your life and embody how you physically would feel if these areas of congestion could be liberated. Open your eyes and write the first thoughts that come to mind.

Dry-brushing will naturally address circulation and the lymphatic system, so don't skip this part of your *dinacharya*. Spend some extra time on the areas of your body where you have a higher concentration of lymph nodes, including your groin, abdomen, chest, underarms, and neck. If you choose to do *abhyanga* (see pages 72–74) after dry-brushing, lean toward more kapha-pacifying oils, such as mustard seed, sesame seed, or mahanarayan oil to help invigorate and circulate.

HA KRIYA (2 MINUTES)

A *kriya* is a technique involving a series of actions aimed at achieving a specific result, often related to energy. In this case, it is a repetitive movement coupled with the sound "ha" to circulate stagnant energy within the body.

For this kriya, stand with your feet wider than your hips. Bend your knees to create muscular activation in your legs. Reach your arms overhead as you inhale, and with a forceful "ha" sound as you exhale, quickly bend your elbows and pull your arms back down. Repeat this eight times. Then in a continuous and similar fashion, reach your arms straight out in front of you as you inhale, and with a sharp "ha" sound, exhale and pull your arms back toward your chest. Repeat this eight times. You'll repeat the cycle, reaching your arms up then forward, on a count of four, then in twos, and then alternating singles for a count of eight. When you complete this, stand with your feet wider than your hips, legs straight and slightly turned in, and move into a forward bend. Stay for three breaths, then slowly push down through your feet to return back to standing.

Midday Rituals

Just as a bellows would fan a fire, "bellows breath" or *bhastrika* generates heat and circulation in the body. As the abdomen is filled with air and then pushed into the lungs, this breathwork promotes alertness of the mind and vitality of the body, generates heat and improves circulation, and promotes an overall clearing effect. Avoid this practice if you are pregnant or have high blood pressure, or if the practice makes you feel panicked or dizzy.

It's ideal to practice bellows breath in a seated position with your hips slightly elevated on a bolster or blanket. You want to be upright, yet have a relaxed feeling across your abdomen so that you'll be able to properly fill and empty. Close your eyes. Breathe as you would naturally, but start to make your breath fuller and deeper. On an exhale, use the contraction of your abdomen to forcefully exhale through the mouth, but without strain. Then, inhale through your nose by expanding your abdomen as your respiratory diaphragm moves downward. This will also have an element of force, but not strain. A full breath may take two to three seconds, and should be at a pace in which the inhale and exhale are the same duration and can be maintained as such. Continue to breathe this way for seven to ten breaths. As you finish, remain seated, observing the way stagnant energy has released and is now circulating in your being.

Red foods are known to have strong lymph-moving properties, and many of these same foods have strong detoxifying abilities. This recipe uses two famously red foods: cherries and beets. Beets are especially proficient at keeping your digestive tract clear, and when ingested along with ground ginger, which delivers a light, drying, and heating punch, you're sure to be free of any lymphatic congestion.

1 cup (240 ml) cherry juice
1 cup (240 ml) beet juice
Pinch of ground ginger
Optional medicinal herb boost: ½ teaspoon manjistha powder

Stir the cherry and beet juice with ½ cup (120 ml) water in a glass and drink at room temperature. If you're using the manjistha powder, it may not dissolve well. One option is to make an herbal infusion by adding the manjistha powder to ½ cup (120 ml) hot water (using this instead of the ½ cup of room temperature water). Let it steep for five minutes, then strain. Stir in the beet and cherry juice and drink at room temperature.

You can help your body do its own work by adding foods and spices that support the lymphatic system into your diet. Incorporate more blueberries, cherries, beets, cranberries, pomegranates, turmeric, leafy green veggies, and seaweed. Don't have these foods exclusively, but make sure that they make a daily appearance.

Evening Rituals

Useful for so many purposes, legs up the wall or *viparita karani* is a restorative yoga posture that places you in a passive and restful inverted position. By elevating your legs and feet above your heart, you are allowing any excess fluid that has accumulated in your legs to move from your lower body toward your abdomen and heart through the lymphatic channels.

Clear enough space at a wall for your legs to extend vertically. If you lack wall space, you can also lie down on your back and with your knees bent, drape your legs over the seat of a chair or couch. When using a wall, lie on your side with your knees pulled in toward your chest and your sitting bones completely up against the wall. Then as you roll onto your back, lift your legs straight up against the wall. This will place you at a 90-degree angle at your hips. Your arms can rest comfortably out from your sides with your palms facing up, or bend your elbows to 90 degrees, like a cactus or goal-post arms. If you're unable to both relax your legs *and* keep them straight, you can either move away from the wall or place a folded blanket under your pelvis to create more space and decrease the tension at the back of your legs. Stay in this posture for at least three minutes and up to ten. When you are ready to come out, bend your knees to your chest and roll to your side.

This massage can either be done as you practice "legs up the wall," or you can do it as a stand-alone exercise afterward. If you choose to do it separately, lie on your back and position your legs in a slightly elevated position. This can be done with pillows, or you could lie on the floor and place your legs over the seat of a couch or a chair. Slightly elevate your head and shoulders to create a natural flow toward the center of your body. Take three deep breaths. Place the palm of one hand slightly below your xiphoid process (the point at the bottom of your sternum), and using very minimal pressure, rub in a clockwise circle twenty times. Then, using only enough pressure to compress your skin, create a pumping action to the rhythm of one pump per every one to two seconds. Do this twenty times. Now, using one hand on each side, position your hands so that they are just below your ribcage, palms down. Angle your hands so they are similar to the angle of your ribs, and begin this same rhythmic pumping twenty times. From your ribcage, move your hands to the inside of your pelvic bone near the crease of each hip. Angle your hands so your fingers point toward your pubic bone. Repeat the light pumping another twenty times. From here, rewind. Go back to the space below your ribcage for twenty pumps, to the gentle pump below your xiphoid for twenty more, and ending with twenty clockwise circles. When complete, rest with your palms up and breathe deeply.

As discussed in the rituals for digestion (pages 195–202), lying on your left side helps to filter waste, including improved movement of lymph. Since our body filters blood through the liver, which is on the right side of the body, sleeping on your left side keeps a steady flow going, preventing blood from getting congested at your liver. Use a pillow to cushion your neck, head, and between your knees to support your muscles on the right side as you sleep.

Seasonal Allergies

Aside from some of the more severe cases, most allergies relate to our body's ability to process what we are taking in. When we are unable to break something down well, it starts to build in our body and to form ama. At this point, your body will signal you in any way it can to stay away from this allergen. Seasonal allergies, such as to tree pollen, ragweed, or mold, are from particles that are airborne, but they aren't so different from food allergies—our body still must be able to digest and eliminate what we are breathing in.

Like many of the conditions we have discussed so far, "allergies" is an umbrella term for a condition that can be expressed through a variety of different symptoms, depending on the season, the person, or other factors, such as diet. If you experience dry eyes, a scratchy throat, or a clear runny nose, this is most likely related to an abundance of air element or vata. Burning sensations or skin sensitivities are an indicator of elevated pitta or fire element. Congestion, more mucus production, or a productive cough signify kapha or the earth element. While you may want to go about addressing them in ways that correspond to the imbalanced dosha, the rituals provided below are excellent for boosting general respiratory health and preventing allergens from being a problem in the first place.

Morning Rituals

RINSE YOUR EYES (3 MINUTES) (SEE PAGE 63)
Don't skip this step in your morning routine if you suffer from seasonal allergies. As your body goes through its nightly cleansing cycle, you'll find little deposits in the corners of your eyes. This amount will be greater if you've been exposed to pollen or other environmental allergens, so it's essential you take the last step to rinse them away. For this purpose, rose or cucumber hydrosol will be most soothing.

As a part of your morning routine, choose to use either a neti pot (see chapter 5) to flush your sinuses, or nasya oil (see pages 69–71) to lubricate them. A neti pot is helpful after spending time outdoors or breathing in polluted air, while nasya is best when your sinuses are feeling dry and irritated.

Not only does this breathing practice create a light and clearing effect that can be a relief when you feel bogged down with the congestion of allergies, but also it stokes your agni. Oftentimes with allergies, even the kind that we breathe in, our digestive fire isn't strong enough to process the allergens. Practices like this can help.

Midday Rituals

ALLERGY-FREE TEA (5 MINUTES)

Counterintuitive as it may sound, honey and bee pollen have properties that can clear away congestion or allergens that have settled into your system; local varieties can be even more beneficial, as they can help build your immunity to seasonal allergens in your area. You'll amplify the effects of this drink by adding *tulsi*, which has an affinity for the respiratory system and is known to clear up even the worst congestion and cough.

1 teaspoon local bee pollen

1 teaspoon tulsi

Optional medicinal herb boost: ½–1 teaspoon nettle leaves or nettle tea

2 cups (480 ml) hot (not boiling) filtered water

1 teaspoon local honey

Place the bee pollen, tulsi, and nettle (if using) in a tea infuser in the water. Steep for ten minutes. Remove the infuser and stir in the honey.

A great midday release, camel pose is good for keeping your heart space open, releasing your chest muscles, and relieving fullness in your chest from colds, other viruses, and allergies. Practice this in an upright kneeling position, padding your knees with a mat, blanket, or towel if necessary. Keeping your hips over your knees, place your hands at the top of your pelvis. Avoid placing them on your lower back so that you do not create an undue amount of bend in your lumbar spine. Your goal is to create a bend through the upper part of your back, or your thoracic spine, and you'll do this by rolling/drawing your shoulders back and lifting your sternum up. Your hands traction your pelvis downward, creating the feeling of your ribcage and pelvis moving in opposite directions. Gaze forward, or you can have a slight tuck with your chin, to ensure you don't overextend your neck. Breathe five deep breaths, inhaling in a way that is most expansive across your chest. Slowly come up by engaging your abdominal muscles, then move to your hands and knees. Gently create a snake-like motion with your spine.

Evening Rituals

HERBAL STEAM (25 MINUTES)

An herbal steam can be the saving grace when you feel like you're so congested that you can't breathe. While there are different over-the-counter remedies that can be effective in clearing congestion, too, those are often drying, not only to your sinuses but to your whole body. The hydration, heat, and herbs make a steam superior to those remedies.

Start your steam by bringing 4 cups (960 ml) water to boil in a large pot. Remove from the heat and add 1 cup (25 g) chamomile or dried chamomile flowers (see Glossary of Herbs, page 267). Cover and let it steep for twenty minutes. Remove the lid, and with a towel draped over your head to trap the steam, place your head over the pot and breathe. Keep taking deep breaths through your nose until you feel that the steam is gone or your congestion has cleared.

OIL EYES (3 MINUTES)

With allergies come dry, inflamed, and irritated eyes. Improve your overall eye health while you soothe your eyes by using castor oil—organic and cold-pressed, if possible—in your eyes at night. Using a dropper that has been cleaned thoroughly with hot, soapy water, administer one to two drops into each eye. Blink a few times, then close your eye for a few minutes to let the oil be distributed. This will blur your vision slightly, so only do this before you go to bed.

Travel

All travel is vata-aggravating because it involves movement and change. There will always be an increase in the air element, but much more if you choose to travel by plane. So in addition to travel jolting your normal routine into jet lag, it's typical to experience vata imbalances like dry skin, constipation, anxiety, joint aches and pains, and insomnia.

We each have our own relationship with travel, and some of us can endure it better than others. No matter where you are on the spectrum, these travel rituals can be useful because the small imbalances that accumulate over time into bigger ones may not be noticeable right away, especially if you travel often (for work or pleasure).

Morning Rituals

SLEEP IN THE ZONE

When traveling on trips shorter than a week and in time zones within three hours of your home, keep your sleep schedule close to normal zone. This will prevent you from experiencing jet lag and make reintegration into your normal schedule much easier. For trips that are either longer than a week or in time zones more than three hours different than your home time zone, adjust to the clock of your destination as soon as possible by sleeping at nightfall and avoiding naps.

MAKE YOURSELF AT HOME (5 MINUTES)

Even if traveling is among your favorite things to do, it's still good to have a home base. No matter the length of your trip, bring elements of home with you. These can be general items that you use for hygiene and self-care, but also consider bringing some items of comfort, such as a photo of your family, a favorite T-shirt, or a scented travel candle that reminds you of home. When you arrive, take some time to designate a space in your room as your travel altar, or to simply arrange these things in a tidy way so that they can be available to you as you need them. While it may take up some extra space in your luggage, having a piece of home with you will keep you settled and grounded when you are away.

Midday Rituals

VICTORIOUS BREATH (UJJAYI BREATHING) (3 MINUTES)

With its ocean-like sound, this breathing practice can soothe and calm you in the same way we can be calmed by white noise. This is useful if you find yourself with anxiety over some turbulence or if being out of your normal home routine has left you unsettled. You can be seated or standing, but it is best when you are able to close your eyes. For this practice, keep your mouth closed without clenching your jaw or tightening your face. Breathe slowly in and out through your nose, making a sound similar to the way you breathe to fog up a mirror or a window—only with your mouth closed. As you inhale, feel your breath move up from your lungs and into your throat. Create a slight constriction at your throat as if to slow the breath, creating a soft "ha" sound. Do this same thing as you exhale. Don't try too hard to create a sound; let it come naturally and without force. Breathe this way for one minute.

CHEW FENNEL SEEDS (1 MINUTE)

Constipation or irregular digestion typically associated with vata imbalance is common when you travel. Fennel seeds are a great digestive herb that are easy to pack in a small container to take along with you. After your lunch, or any time you feel like you have bloating or indigestion, take a pinch of fennel seeds (approximately five seeds), chew them completely, and swallow them. If you find that they are too fibrous to swallow, you can also chew them for several minutes to release the medicinal oils and then spit them out.

The best food choices for travel are both vata-pacifying and easy to process. Sitting in a car or an airplane can make you feel stagnant, so you may crave something light and fresh like fruit or a salad. Entertain this craving, but make the majority of your choices on the first one to two days grounding and easy to digest. Think soup, stews, cooked veggies, and white rice, and do your best to stick to meal times and avoid snacking, as it can disrupt your digestive cycle. And while traveling, particularly for pleasure, it can be tempting to indulge in foods you may not typically eat. It isn't necessary to be so rigid that you don't enjoy local cuisine or have a few decadent treats, but know that your digestion will be happiest when you consume familiar foods for the majority of your trip.

Evening Rituals

GARLAND POSE (MALASANA) (3 MINUTES)

This deep squat can feel challenging to our chair-bound society but it assists our digestion and grounds our nervous system. While in comfortable clothing and without wearing your shoes, place your feet slightly wider than your hips. Turn out your feet in a comfortable angle and begin to bend your knees, making sure they move in the same direction as your toes. Your aim is to squat as low as you can or to a full bend at your knees and hips, so that as your hands are placed together at your sternum, your elbows press out into your thighs. Lengthen up through your spine as your hips move down. Breathe ten deep breaths in the squat. Either return to standing and gently move your hips in a circle and bend your knees to release your legs, or release your hands to the floor and fold forward in a wide-leg forward bend (see page 162).

The tremendous amount of bend required by your knees and hips in malasana may call for a modification. If your heels lift, simply roll a blanket up and slide it underneath them. This also works if you find it difficult to elongate your spine. If it seems nearly impossible to get into this shape, try mimicking the position on your back. Lie back and bring your knees toward the outsides of your ribcage with your hands at your shins or at the backs of your thighs. Let your pelvis, lower back, and shoulders rest heavy on the floor. Breathe ten slow, deep breaths and then release.

GROUNDING MEDITATION (5 MINUTES)

It can be difficult to stick to a meditation practice when you are on the road. Scheduling time to be still, along with keeping your room organized and clean, can be helpful. Additionally, if you brought some personal items with you to remind you of home, you can set them up as a temporary altar (see page 116). You can choose to continue your regular meditation practice, or consider one geared toward keeping you rooted when travel feels unsettling.

Sit upright on the floor in a way that feels supported and where it is possible for you to lengthen your spine. Place a blanket over your shoulders, and wrap it around the front of your body, using the blanket both for its heavy, grounding quality and to create a cocoon. Keeping your arms inside the blanket wrap, let your palms rest face up on your lap. With your eyes closed, inhale and say to yourself, "I am grounded." Exhale and say, "I am calm." Continue this practice for five minutes.

Weakened Immunity or Low Ojas

We all know that a strong immune system is important for staying healthy, especially in times of stress. *Ojas* is our vitality or an essence, that is very similar to our immunity. It's what makes someone radiant glowingand keeps them in good health, so that they can pursue the things in life that make them thrive. Our ojas can become low if we don't get enough sleep, have weak digestion, eat poorly, work too much, or don't allow time for people and things that feed our soul. During those times, we are more susceptible to illnesses. Note that adrenal fatigue (page 163) and burnout (page 182) are two conditions of low ojas.

When I was fifteen, I had a moped so I could navigate around my small town without having to rely on my parents. It had two fuel tanks: a main tank and a reserve tank. If I got low on fuel, I could flip a switch from main to reserve to help get me to the nearest gas station. Ojas is like this reserve tank. You want to keep it full in case there is an emergency, but better if you can get along without using it. Signs of lowered immunity or low ojas can appear before your main fuel tank is empty, but longer recovery is needed if you've gone through your primary fuel source and started depleting your energy stores.

Ojas can be rebuilt through specific herbs and foods, spending time with loved ones, regular *abhyanga*, and resting. Thus, even though there may be various reasons that your immunity and vitality have decreased, we can follow a common path to restoration. In these rituals you'll see a general theme for resting and slowing down, with an overall focus on rebuilding.

Morning Rituals

Even before almond milk became a trend, people practicing Ayurveda were using it as a DIY healing tonic. Store-bought almond milk can still have a stellar nutritional profile, but when you're using it to rebuild ojas, what you make at home can't be replaced. Almonds are said to have an affinity for ojas and when you make them into a milk, you are bringing the essence of the healing properties into a more digestible and concentrated form. Many people assume making your own almond milk is time-consuming or a daunting task, but it really takes less than ten minutes and has minimal cleanup. Drink one cup of this homemade recipe every night. Sprinkle with fresh nutmeg for extra calming effects.

Makes 4 cups (960 ml) or 4 servings

>1 cup (85 g) raw almonds, soaked overnight in room-temperature filtered water
>
>½ teaspoon sea salt
>
>1 teaspoon vanilla bean powder or ½ teaspoon vanilla extract (optional)
>
>2 dates, pitted and soaked for 5–10 minutes (optional)
>
>Optional medicinal herb boost: 1 teaspoon chyavanprash

1. Drain the almonds and add them to a blender with the salt, vanilla (if using), and dates. Add the chyavanprash, if using.
2. Add 4 cups (960 ml) filtered water and blend until creamy, 2 to 3 minutes.
3. Strain with cheesecloth (by placing it over a large bowl) or a fine-mesh strainer. Squeeze or press until all of the liquid has come out. The remaining pulp can be saved for other uses (for example, dried and as flour for baking), or it can be composted or discarded.
4. Store the almond milk in an airtight container or bottle in the refrigerator for up to five days.

MEDITATION FOR RESTORING AND REBUILDING (5 MINUTES)

Your thoughts may be your strongest asset for restoration. Use this meditation to create an inner framework that supports you in rebuilding your immunity and ojas. This meditation can be practiced seated with your palms facing up, or you can try it standing in what feels like a power stance, by placing your feet slightly wider than your hips, bending your knees slightly, and holding your hands palms-up at your sides. Close your eyes and begin to breathe deeply, using a slow and methodical breath. Now, bring attention to an area of your life where you have felt weak or inadequate. What are the descriptors of this? Is it that you feel financially unstable, underprepared for your job, or just not enough? Create a mantra by using one to three sentences that represent you being strong in these aspects, such as, "My life is abundant. I am ready for what may come. I am enough." Repeat these phrases to yourself, imagining your evolution in these areas, going from weak to strong. After three to five minutes, slowly open your eyes and see things from your new perspective.

Midday Rituals

BALANCED BREATHING (SAMA VRITTI) (3 MINUTES) (SEE PAGE 206)

As you work to boost your immunity, the steady quality of balanced breathing can help. When you finish this practice, take time to pause and observe how your entire being feels. Recognize this as a baseline that you can return to if the day becomes trying.

NASYA (3 MINUTES) (SEE PAGES 69–71)

Nourishing your nervous system shouldn't be overlooked when our interest is in becoming stronger in both the body and the mind. Nasya is the quickest and most efficient way to supply your brain with healing oils and herbs. It can also serve as a natural pick-me-up in the middle of the day.

Evening Rituals

When you feel weak, low, fatigued, or sick, it is easy to fall into a storyline that you think was meant to be your own. When this happens, you might create an inner monologue around this story, perpetuating the cycle. But *you* are the author of your own story, which means you can change it. Use these journal prompts to make a shift in your thinking and to live out your favorite story.

How do you feel now?
What phrases do you tell yourself or others that feed into your current story?
How do you want to feel?
What are the phrases you will use with your new story?
How did you contribute to your ideal story today?
How will you contribute to your ideal story tomorrow?

This is one of the most calming and comforting yoga poses. It creates a feeling of being held and taken care of, and with the extra support from blankets, you'll feel like you've gone back to the womb. To practice, you'll need a yoga bolster and a blanket, or several blankets (a stack about 6 to 8 inches/15 to 20 cm high) folded lengthwise to match the length of your torso. Start in a kneeling position, with your feet touching and your knees wide. Slide your bolster between your knees so that the length extends away from you. Fold forward from your hips, letting your torso stretch out across the bolster. Place another blanket, across your lower back and pelvis—or cover your entire body with a blanket (it helps to have an assistant)—using the weight to create an ultimate grounding effect. Choose either to place your arms along your body with your head resting and turned to one side, or to stack your hands on the bolster and place your forehead on your hands. Breathe naturally as you stay in position for three to five minutes. When you're ready to come out of the posture, move slowly, letting your head be the last thing to lift.

The End Cycle

I admittedly took my first yoga class because what I had seen in pictures looked like gymnastics for adults, and I'm someone who is intrigued by movement, so this appealed to me. I left my first class feeling more aware, like my senses had been heightened. The music in my car seemed louder and people seemed to be moving faster, when all I wanted was to slow down and turn inward. The practice felt intentional and I suddenly felt a need to live my life more intentionally, too. I knew I had started down a path and I was unlikely to turn back.

For me, studying Ayurveda added a new and vital layer to the idea of living with intention. From the color clothes I was wearing to the temperature of the water I was drinking to whether I participated in small talk, nothing was arbitrary anymore. The more mindful I was of my decisions, the more meaningful my life became—I started living as my true authentic self. There was less questioning if I was doing things right, and more checking in to see if I was doing things right for *me* in any given moment.

As a part of this process, I found it more necessary to shape my everyday routines so they could provide a foundation for who I am and a means for carrying out life the way I want to live it. At times, this could mean weaving in something new to make me feel better, and at other times, a rediscovery of something that makes me feel alive. Nature is always the common denominator; going back to my childhood, I knew in my body that seeking harmony between the nature within us and that which surrounds us leads to our ultimate well-being. I see, listen, and learn from nature. I understand how the sweet taste of fresh berries in the summer can be as joyful as days spent at the pool as a kid. And that there is no hierarchy of the seasons. Those summer days that are full of energy are no more important than the restful days of winter. Every season and element has its role.

Though nature moves and changes on its own terms, we get to decide how nature will affect us. Every day, it's our choice to look both within ourselves and beyond ourselves, tuning into our individual needs and what nature is offering to fulfill them. We can either continue down a path that doesn't lead to where we want to go, or we can be patient with ourselves as we learn to break the old cycles, leaving space for new and improved ones to begin. Use what you have learned from this book—about yourself, nature, and Ayurveda—as a tool of empowerment so that you, too, can create rituals and routines in your life, to live as your healthiest and truest self.

Ritual Journaling

The things we choose to better ourselves with won't work if we aren't able to properly integrate them. Allowing adequate time for their completion, making sure our goals are realistic, and giving ourselves a pat on the back for showing up and trying even if we don't always succeed, are all ways we can have better follow-through with our intentions. Sometimes, the right tool is all we need to make us more consistent and effective.

This journal format was designed to help you do exactly that. Whether it is something you are using to get started or is an ongoing part of your routine, it will help you seamlessly weave healthy rituals into your day and evening.

The prompts below are geared toward creating a mindful opening and closing to your day, along with space for self-reflection. Unlike other journals, this isn't a place for your to-do list; to keep things feeling ritualistic, it could be worth the investment of a new journal and pen.

You'll find three different templates for journaling. First, there's a place to establish what your rituals will be for the week, including the reasons why they are important to you at this time. The next is a daily record of whether or not you've been able to complete your rituals, along with notes on your success and where you could use some encouragement. Lastly, there is a section for recording your weekly reflections. This information will help you plan your rituals accordingly for the weeks to come.

Rearranging your day isn't easy, so reread chapters 8 and 9 before you begin, and consider those tips for building new and effective rituals.

Weekly Journal

At the beginning of the week, establish up to three rituals that you would like to do every morning, midday, and evening. Add a time estimate to ensure you are being realistic in your endeavor, and make a personal note as to why these rituals are especially important to you.

Week of January 1

MY MORNING WELLNESS RITUAL

1. Meditation   Time Required *10 min.*

2. Drink hot lemon water   Time Required *5 min.*

3. Oil massage/abhyanga   Time Required *20 min.*

Total time required to conduct entire morning ritual in a mindful manner is *35 min.*

I choose this morning ritual because *I've been feeling low energy and my days have felt rushed and unfulfilled.*

When I complete this morning ritual, I (will) feel *like I have more control over my day and that I can be fully present with people and make conscious decisions.*

MY MIDDAY WELLNESS RITUAL

1. Take a walk around the block   Time Required *5 min.*

2. Breathe 3 deep breaths   Time Required *1 min.*

3. Sit for 3 minutes with my eyes closed   Time Required *3 min.*

Total time required to conduct entire midday ritual in a mindful manner is *9 min.*

I choose this midday ritual because *I get tired in the afternoon and often begin to lose focus.*

When I complete this midday ritual, I (will) feel *rested, rejuvenated, and energized to finished the day.*

MY EVENING WELLNESS RITUAL

1. Make nightly sleep elixir   Time Required *10 min.*

2. Oil my feet   Time Required *5 min.*

3. Breathing exercises   Time Required *5 min.*

Total time required to conduct entire evening ritual in a mindful manner is *20 min.*

I choose this evening ritual because *I have been waking up during the night, so in the morning I don't feel rested.*

When I complete this evening ritual, *I (will) feel like I can go to bed with a clear mind and don't have difficulty getting to sleep or staying asleep. It makes me feel like my day has a gentle, rather than abrupt, ending.*

Daily Journal

Every day, check off the rituals you've completed. Write about the empowering feelings that you had so that when you look back, either for inspiration or motivation, you can recall the impact these actions had. And because there is always a possibility that things aren't going as you had planned, list the things that can create a more supportive and encouraging environment for you.

Day 1 January 1

- ☐ Morning Ritual
- ☐ Midday Ritual
- ☐ Evening Ritual

I had more energy in the afternoon and was able to exercise after work. I didn't feel anxious when things didn't go as planned. I felt like I had more time for work and family, despite taking extra time to care for myself.

It's difficult to get to bed at the time I should for the proper amount of sleep. The evening feels like the only "me time" in my day, and I'm often not ready for bed despite being tired.

Weekly Reflection

Yes, with the exception of morning abhyanga. All of the rituals were easy to integrate, but abhyanga takes longer and I found myself feeling rushed in the morning.

Change my full abhyanga to oiling just my neck, hips, and lower back since these areas seem to hold stress tension and hurt at the end of the day. This will take less time. I'm also traveling next week, so I need to remember to pack my ritual supplies.

Weekly Journal

Sample pages

Week of ___ / ___ / ___

MY MORNING WELLNESS RITUAL

1. _____   Time Required _____

2. _____   Time Required _____

3. _____   Time Required _____

Total time required to conduct entire morning ritual in a mindful manner is _____ .

I choose this morning ritual because _____

_____ .

When I complete this morning ritual, I (will) feel _____

_____ .

MY MIDDAY WELLNESS RITUAL

1. _____   Time Required _____

2. _____   Time Required _____

3. _____   Time Required _____

Total time required to conduct entire midday ritual in a mindful manner is _____ .

I choose this midday ritual because

.

When I complete this midday ritual, I (will) feel

.

1. _____   Time Required

2. _____   Time Required

3. _____   Time Required

Total time required to conduct entire evening ritual in a mindful manner is   .

I choose this evening ritual because

.

When I complete this evening ritual, I (will) feel

.

Daily Journal

Sample pages

Day 1 ___ /___ /___

- ☐ Morning Ritual
- ☐ Midday Ritual
- ☐ Evening Ritual

THINGS THAT FELT EMPOWERING TODAY:

.

AREAS WHERE I COULD USE ENCOURAGEMENT:

.

Day 2 ___ /___ /___

- ☐ Morning Ritual
- ☐ Midday Ritual
- ☐ Evening Ritual

THINGS THAT FELT EMPOWERING TODAY:

.

AREAS WHERE I COULD USE ENCOURAGEMENT:

.

Day 3 ___ /___ /___

☐ Morning Ritual

☐ Midday Ritual

☐ Evening Ritual

THINGS THAT FELT EMPOWERING TODAY:

.

AREAS WHERE I COULD USE ENCOURAGEMENT:

.

Day 4 ___ /___ /___

☐ Morning Ritual

☐ Midday Ritual

☐ Evening Ritual

THINGS THAT FELT EMPOWERING TODAY:

AREAS WHERE I COULD USE ENCOURAGEMENT:

Day 5 ___ /___ /___

☐ Morning Ritual

☐ Midday Ritual

☐ Evening Ritual

THINGS THAT FELT EMPOWERING TODAY:

Day 6 ___ / ___ / ___

- ☐ Morning Ritual
- ☐ Midday Ritual
- ☐ Evening Ritual

Day 7 ___ / ___ / ___

- ☐ Morning Ritual
- ☐ Midday Ritual
- ☐ Evening Ritual

THINGS THAT FELT EMPOWERING TODAY:

_____

_____ .

AREAS WHERE I COULD USE ENCOURAGEMENT:

_____

_____ .

Weekly Reflection

Sample pages

WAS I REALISTIC IN PLANNING MY RITUALS?

_____

_____

_____

_____ .

SHOULD MODIFICATIONS BE MADE FOR NEXT WEEK?

_____

_____

_____

_____ .

Resources

Ancient Organics   ancientorganics.com
Organic ghee made using traditional Ayurvedic methods

The Art of Living Retreat Center   artoflivingretreatcenter.org
Ayurvedic spa and panchakarma center

The Ayurvedic Institute   ayurveda.com
An Ayurvedic school with a website that includes articles,
recipes, and Ayurvedic products

Banyan Botanicals   banyanbotanicals.com
Ayurvedic herbs, oils, supplies, and informational resources

California College of Ayurveda   ayurvedacollege.com
An Ayurvedic school with a website that contains resources and
educational articles

Chandika   chandika.com
Ayurvedic products ranging from herbs to skincare

The Chopra Center   chopra.com
An Ayurvedic spa with an informational website that includes
online courses and self-care products

Diamond Way Ayurveda   diamondwayayurveda.com

A unique offering of books and products for Ayurvedic skincare and bodywork

Hale Pule   halepule.com

A center for Ayurvedic courses and yoga courses alike, in person and online

Joyful Belly   joyfulbelly.com

Resource for Ayurvedic recipes, remedies, and certification programs

LifeSpa   lifespa.com

Ayurvedic herbs, oils, supplies, informational resources, and a treatment center

Manduka   manduka.com

Yoga supplies, such as mats, bolsters, blocks, and straps

Mount Madonna Institute   mountmadonna.org

A retreat center and school with Ayurveda programs and other spiritual courses

Mountain Rose Herbs   mountainroseherbs.com

Organic, fair-trade herbs, spices, oils, and plant waters or hydrosols

National Ayurvedic Medicine Association   ayurvedanama.org

Association supporting education and the professional practice of Ayurveda; includes locator for an Ayurvedic practitioner near you

Pukka Herbs   pukkaherbs.us

Teas and herbs inspired by Ayurveda

Pratima Spa and Skincare   pratimaskincare.com

Ayurvedic skincare products, informational resources, and a day spa

The Raj   theraj.com

Ayurvedic hotel, spa, and treatment center

Sarada Ayurvedic Remedies   saradausa.com

Ayurvedic oils for the body and skincare made using traditional formulas

Starwest Botanicals   starwest-botanicals.com

Organic and fair-trade herbs, spices, and essential oils

Surya Spa   suryaspa.com

Authentic Ayurvedic clinic offering consultations and traditional treatments

Glossary of Herbs

Herbal therapies are wonderful in that they assit our bodies in regulating functions, instead of serving as a replacement for the function. This means we aren't likely to become dependent upon them, and we can ultimately stop taking an herb once we are feeling better. Like prescription medications, there can be contraindications or potential side effects; yet herbal side effects are typically very mild and go away as soon as you stop taking the herb.

This list of herbs includes all the culinary spices and medicinal herbs from the recipes and rituals in this book, but there are many others that are also widely used by Ayurvedic practitioners which are not included here. Herbs have specific actions and an affinity for certain systems of the body. An herb may be appealing to you for a specific use, but you must be aware that that is not its only use. Without this knowledge, you may end up either taking something that will be ineffective for you, or help one thing while provoking another.

While this glossary is meant to help you understand more about the recipes and why they were chosen for each condition, this glossary should not act as a stand in for advice you receive from your Ayurvedic practitioner or other healthcare provider.

How to Interpret and Use This Glossary

Dosha: This tells you which doshas can benefit from taking the herb by using a (−) sign to note that it is pacifying. It will cause aggravation if you see a (+) sign. If you see a (=), this means it is neutral and neither increases nor decreases the dosha.

Energy: The energy refers to the thermal effect of the herb, or if it creates heat or cold in the body.

Gunas: These are the most notable gunas or qualities of the herb. Though twenty gunas are discussed to describe the elements and doshas (see page 15), there are five primary gunas used for describing herbal energetics: light, which has a reducing action on tissue; heavy, which builds and nourishes tissue; oily, which is unctuous and can coat surfaces; dry which absorbs moisture and reduces tissue; and sharp, which penetrates tissue quickly.

Contraindications: These are the exceptions and circumstances when you should not consume the herb. It is always recommended that you speak with your healthcare practitioner prior to taking herbs, especially if you have a current health condition or are taking another medication.

ALOE
Dosha: V=P=K=
Energy: Cooling
Gunas: Heavy, oily
Contraindications: Pregnancy
Aloe is a female reproductive tonic and can be especially useful for those experiencing excessive bleeding, clotting, or symptoms of menopause. It's healing for inflammatory conditions of the skin. It's also effective in treating

inflammatory conditions of the gastrointestinal tract, such as ulcerative colitis, ulcers, or hyperacidity.

Dosha: V=P–K–
Energy: Cooling
Gunas: Light, dry
Contraindications: Pregnancy, constipation

If you're familiar with the yogic text the Bhagavad Gita, you'll recognize Arjuna as the name of the hero of the story. The herb is well-known for its heart health properties, ranging from decreasing hypertension to reducing congestive heart conditions to healing a broken heart. It is also useful for alleviating respiratory conditions, such as asthma and bronchitis, and can be helpful in promoting wound healing and inflammatory conditions of the skin.

Dosha: V–P+K–
Energy: Heating
Gunas: Light, oily
Contraindications: High pitta/high heat conditions or excess ama

Ashwagandha is an adaptogen, meaning it plays a supportive role during stressful times. It can help to regulate the nervous system and act as either a sedative or a nerve tonic. It's rejuvenating for muscle tissue and aids in rebuilding all tissues in the case of emaciation or other debilitating conditions. This herb has an affinity for the male reproductive system and can promote fertility and libido, but it is also good for women and treating female reproductive deficiencies. Ashwagandha can also be used in treating the thyroid.

Dosha: V–P–K=
Energy: Cooling
Gunas: Light, dry
Contraindications: Constipation

Bhringaraj has an affinity for our head—both for healing physical ailments, such as hearing problems, vertigo, and sinus issues, and for soothing mental agitation that arises with stress in particular. It's best known as a hair tonic and for reversing graying and baldness. It's a calming herb that can be used for sleep, but it also has other uses, such as treating inflammatory skin conditions, liver problems, and conditions of the lungs.

BRAHMI

Dosha: V=P=K=
Energy: Cooling
Gunas: Light
Contraindications: None known

Brahmi's claim to fame is its effects on the nervous system. It's used as a brain tonic for improving memory and learning disabilities, along with conditions of the mind that come with stress. It's used as a nerve tonic in treating Parkinson's, Alzheimer's, and dementia, in addition to treating skin conditions where the nervous system is the underlying cause.

BOSWELLIA

Dosha: V–P–K–
Energy: Heating and cooling
Gunas: Light, dry, sharp
Contraindications: Pregnancy

Boswellia is also known as Indian frankincense, and it has a unique quality in that it can be heating and cooling at the same time. It can help to increase circulation while simultaneously decreasing inflammation, making it great for pain or inflammatory conditions, especially of the joints. It is exceptional for preventing hard scar tissue or dense fascial tissue from forming, reducing changes in tissue composition that can limit joint mobility. Many use this for its spiritual connection, either as an essential oil or incense, as it is said to open the mind.

CARDAMOM

Dosha: V–P–K–
Energy: Cooling
Gunas: Light, dry
Contraindications: Excess pitta or heat.

When considering digestive aids, one should always put cardamom on the list. It's effective in strengthening digestion and reducing indigestion and gas. It's also helpful for treating morning sickness and other conditions with nausea. Cardamom clears the lungs and heals sore throats, thus making it good for seasonal colds.

CHAMOMILE

Dosha: V+P–K–
Energy: Cooling
Gunas: Light, dry
Contraindications: None known

This flower or herb is commonly prepared as a tea and is widely known for its calming effects. It is relieving of nerve pain, heated digestive conditions, and headaches. For those experiencing difficulty with menstruation, it can be regulating.

CHYAVANPRASH

Dosha: V=P=K=
Energy: Heating
Gunas: Heavy
Contraindications: In excess, can be too heating for pitta dosha

Chyavanprash is a jam that is made of both medicinal herbs and culinary spices. Some consider this to be Ayurveda's equivalent of a multivitamin in terms of its use. Depending on the recipe, it could have twenty or more ingredients, giving it a myriad of benefits. Among the more common ingredients used are amalaki, ghee, and cardamom. This is used universally to increase vitality and to strengthen immunity, and it is considered rejuvenating to all tissues of the body.

Dosha: V–P+K-
Energy: Healing
Gunas: Light, dry, sharp
Contraindications: Excessive heat in the gastrointestinal tract

This is a spice most have in their kitchen and it has many medicinal uses. Reach for cinnamon when you have a cold or sinus congestion, or when your digestion feels slow or sluggish. Cinnamon can be used to treat colic, diarrhea, and imbalanced intestinal flora. The heat of cinnamon is good for circulation, especially in the case of cold extremities.

Dosha: V–P=K-
Energy: Cooling
Gunas: Light, oily, sharp
Contraindications: Inflammatory conditions

Cloves have been used for years as an antiseptic and numbing agent in dentistry. Usage is not limited to this, as cloves also have a direct effect on digestion by increasing agni without much aggravation of pitta. They're also helpful in treating colds when there is congestion or a sore throat, and reduce muscle and joint pain when used externally.

Dosha: V–P–K-
Energy: Cooling
Gunas: Light, oily
Contraindications: None known

Coriander is popularly used as a digestive remedy in treating irritable bowel syndrome, colic, and inflammatory digestive conditions such as Chron's disease, ulcers or acid reflux. It's a great fever reducer and can clear mucus from the lungs, making it good for seasonal colds and flus. The leaf, or cilantro, it is used externally in treating skin conditions, especially from allergies, and internally for heavy metal detoxification.

Dosha: V=P=K=
Energy: Cooling
Gunas: Light, dry
Contraindications: Use with caution with inflammatory conditions in the digestive tract

The Sanskrit name for cumin is *jiraka*, which means to promote digestion— and that is exactly what this herb is best known rto do. It can help increase the absorption of nutrients when cooking, is a remedy for diarrhea, and decreases indigestion and nausea. It's also used for increasing breast milk production, and for conditions of the lungs, such as chest tightness.

Dosha: V–P=K–
Energy: Heating
Gunas: Heavy, dry
Contraindications: Pregnancy

Dashmula means "ten roots," and this combination of herbs is one of the most grounding formulas one can use. It is often recommended for those experiencing vata (ether or air) imbalances and is a nervine used for pain, sciatica, anxiety, and Parkinson's disease. Dashmula is also used in treating weakness of the immune system.

Dosha: V=P=K=
Energy: Heating (slightly)
Gunas: Light, dry
Contraindications: None known

Fennel is another herb that is classically used for digestion. It relieves discomfort from bloating, cramps, gas, and nausea, and can increase agni without aggravating pitta. It's also used for treating urinary tract conditions, for smooth muscle spasms, and in clearing the respiratory tract.

GINGER

Dosha: V–P+K–
Energy: Heating
Gunas: Fresh root is heavy, oily; dry powder is light, dry, sharp
Contraindications: Conditions of high pitta, such as heartburn, high blood pressure, or inflammatory skin conditions

Ginger is a rhizome or root that has many medicinal uses along with being a household spice. Think of ginger for colds or respiratory illnesses, as it is good for clearing mucus. Use it to increase your digestive fire, to reduce gas, to decrease nausea, and to prevent travel sickness. Ginger can treat joint conditions, including arthritis, as it increases circulation while acting as an anti-inflammatory.

GOTU KOLA

Dosha: V=P–K–
Energy: Cooling
Gunas: Light, dry
Contraindications: Pregnancy

Gotu kola is a blood purifier, nerve rejuvenator, and adaptogenic herb. It supports your body under stress and can help improve memory and alertness. Gotu kola is well-known for its ability to heal inflammatory joint and skin conditions, but it also moonlights as a beauty herb, as it's great for promoting clear skin and lustrous hair.

GUDUCHI

Dosha: V–P–K=
Energy: Heating
Gunas: Light, oily
Contraindications: Pregnancy

Guduchi is a bitter herb and is known to alleviate burning sensations and reduce fevers, while it simultaneously helps support the liver in detoxification. It's used to treat autoimmune diseases by boosting the immune system, and it is great for improving inflammatory skin conditions.

Dosha: V+P–K–
Energy: Cooling
Gunas: Light, dry
Contraindications: Conditions of high vata or excessive cold

Hibiscus is a flower that is purifying to the blood and heart. It's often used in beauty remedies as a way to promote a clear complexion and hair growth. The female reproductive system can benefit from hibiscus, especially in the case of a heavy menstrual cycle.

Dosha: V–P–K–
Energy: Cooling
Gunas: Heavy, oily
Contraindications: High blood pressure, edema, liver disorders, pregnancy

Licorice is a root that is used for many different systems. It benefits the lungs by treating dry and productive coughs, asthma, and bronchitis. Its ability to coat makes it good for sore throats, ulcers, or hyperacidity, where tissue needs soothing. It is used for promoting strength in the adrenal glands and nervous system, and it's good for treating dry or inflammatory skin conditions.

Dosha: V+P–K–
Energy: Cooling
Gunas: Heavy, dry
Contraindications: High vata conditions

Manjistha means "red root" and as red foods do, it helps to treat the lymphatic system. It has an affinity for the skin and can clear eczema, psoriasis, acne, and rosacea. It is used to stop bleeding in conditions such as ulcers and Crohn's disease, and to regulate menstrual cycles.

Dosha: V–P+K–
Energy: Heating
Gunas: Heavy, oily
Contraindications: Congestion

Mucuna pruriens, also called *kapikacchu*, is a nerve tonic. It has a naturally occurring precursor to the neurotransmitter dopamine, which is often deficient in those with depression. It's also a reproductive tonic, working to treat low libido and to improve fertility for both men and women.

Dosha: V–P–K–
Energy: Cooling, heating in excess
Gunas: Light, dry, sharp
Contraindications: Epilepsy, high vata conditions

Mint is another common herb whose taste is familiar, but whose medicinal benefits may be less well-known. It's used in treating colds, as it can produce sweating and clear congestion. It's settling to the nervous system when one is under stress or emotional tension. It's used externally in sprays or ointments for treating inflammatory skin conditions.

Dosha: V–P+K–
Energy: Heating
Gunas: Light, dry, sharp
Contraindications: Inflammatory conditions

Mustard seeds have an affinity for the lungs and joints. They can reduce mucus in the respiratory tract, they aid in breathing for those with bronchitis or pneumonia, and they prevent colds from fully manifesting. In joint conditions, such as arthritis, they are used to regulate pain and swelling.

Dosha: V+P–K–
Energy: Cooling

Gunas: Light, dry

Contraindications: Emaciation or wasting

Neem is the first herb that comes to mind for treating skin. It's used for all inflammatory conditions of the skin and is especially good at healing bacterial and fungal infections, both internally and externally. It's an antiseptic and used for oral hygiene. The cool and bitter qualities make it good for digestive and respiratory conditions associated with high pitta or inflammation.

NETTLE

Dosha: V+P–K–

Energy: Cooling

Gunas: Light, dry

Contraindications: None known

Nettle is an *alterative* or blood cleanser. It is used for treating asthma, mucus in the respiratory tract, and allergies. It is also used as an anti-inflammatory.

NUTMEG

Dosha: V–P+K–

Energy: Heating

Gunas: Light, oily, sharp

Contraindications: Avoid in high doses, i.e., greater than six grams

Nutmeg is a nervine, and as a sedative, it is used to treat insomnia and an overactive mind. In addition to relaxing the mind, it can relax muscles, such as in the case of restless legs syndrome. Use nutmeg to help absorb nutrients in the small intestine and also to help with stomach cramps, pain, or bloating.

ROSE

Dosha: V=P=K=

Energy: Cooling

Gunas: Light, dry

Contraindications: None known

From now on, when you think of rose, think of its ability to calm and clear skin and how it helps treat the female reproductive system. It can be used to alleviate PMS and to decrease symptoms of menopause. As a cooling herb, it is good for treating inflammatory conditions of the digestive tract and is said to help control blood lipid levels.

SAFFRON

Dosha: V–P=K–
Energy: Heating
Gunas: Light, oily
Contraindications: Pregnancy

Saffron has an affinity for the blood, heart, and reproductive system. It's used to regulate menstrual cycles and aid in fertility problems, in addition to being an aphrodisiac. Saffron is also helpful in treating congestive heart conditions and anemia.

SALT

Dosha: V–P+K+
Energy: Heating
Gunas: Heavy, sharp
Contraindications: High blood pressure

There are different types of salt, such as rock salt and sea salt. Rock salt is easier to digest, whereas sea salt has more mineral content. Salt benefits digestion by stimulating our digestive fire and can also help to clear mucus from the lungs.

SHATAVARI

Dosha: V–P–K+
Energy: Cooling
Gunas: Heavy, oily
Contraindications: Low digestive fire

Shatavari is the go-to herb for balancing female hormones. It regulates menstrual cycles, but also helps with fertility, preventing miscarriages, and decreasing hot flashes in menopause. It can be used to treat inflammatory digestive conditions, helps to rebuild tissues when we have lowered immunity, and is also an adaptogenic herb, meaning it helps our body cope with stress.

SKULLCAP

Dosha: V=P–K–
Energy: Cooling
Gunas: Light
Contraindications: None known

Skullcap is used primarily for its nervine effects, such as promoting mental clarity, calming an agitated mind, and reducing insomnia. It is said to be especially good for pitta and for calming pitta emotions.

TRIPHALA

Dosha: V=P=K=
Energy: Cooling
Gunas: Light, dry
Contraindications: None known

Triphala is an herbal formula made of three different fruits: haritaki, amalaki, and bibhitaki. Each fruit is pacifying for a dosha or doshic type of digestion, making it a tridoshic formula. Triphala is one of the first herbs to think of when treating indigestion, as each of the three herbs is proficient in treating the different types of imbalanced agni. It also benefits the skin and eyes by decreasing inflammation.

TULSI

Dosha: V–P+K–
Energy: Heating
Gunas: Light, dry
Contraindications: High pitta conditions

Tulsi is also known as holy basil and is revered as a plant that can create spiritual clarity. Tulsi has an affinity for the lungs, so it is especially useful for treating conditions of the lungs and upper respiratory tract, including asthma, bronchitis, and allergies. Its ability to both treat congestion and reduce fevers makes it useful for remedying colds.

Dosha: V–P–K–

Energy: Heating

Gunas: Light, dry

Contraindications: Avoid high doses during pregnancy or in conjunction with blood thinners

The Sanskrit word for turmeric is *harida*, which means "yellow." The powder this root produces is indeed recognizable for its yellow color, and due to the many research studies touting its medicinal uses, its name has become familiar to many. There is a lengthy list of benefits for this herb and it could almost be assumed that if you have an ailment, turmeric will help. Among its many healing qualities are its anti-inflammatory effect, it ability to increase blood flow, antibiotic properties, and topical uses for cuts and bruises.

Dosha: V–P–K–

Energy: Heating

Gunas: Light, oily

Contraindications: Depression.

This sedating, heavy herb is known to promote sleep. It's warm and grounding and can relieve tension and feelings of restlessness, especially when they are caused by anxiety. Valerian has also been used to help reduce symptoms of withdrawal for those in the process of quitting addictive drugs.

Glossary of Ayurvedic Terms

Abhyanga—oil massage or anointing of oil that is part of an Ayurvedic dinacharya

Agni—the digestive fire that is necessary for processing any physical (food) or non-physical (emotions) thing taken in by the body or senses

Ama—accumulated waste in the body that can't be digested or absorbed

Asana—a posture, or seat, in yoga

Ayurveda—the "science of life;" a traditional medicine from India

Bhuta—element; there are five elements that make up nature (ether, air, fire, water, and earth)

Dhatu—one of seven tissues that support the body, each formed in a sequential way

Dinacharya—Ayurveda's daily routine

Doshas—the three constitutions, vata, pitta, and kapha, that bring health when balanced and sickness when imbalanced

Gandusha—the oral-cleansing practice of oil pulling that is part of an Ayurvedic daily routine

Garshana—the practice of dry-brushing the body, that is part of an Ayurvedic daily routine

Ghee—butter that has had the milk solids removed; also called clarified butter

Guna—an attribute or quality, used to describe the elements and doshas; there are twenty in total

Ida nadi—the main energetic channel on the left side of the body that represents the feminine or lunar energy

Kapha—one of the three doshas; the constitution of earth and water

Nadi—a channel, such as an energy channel or the pulse

Ojas—the vitality that provides for our strength and immunity

Panchakarma—the five actions of cleansing or purification, including vomiting, purgation, enema, administration of oil through the nose, and bloodletting

Pingala nadi—the main energetic channel on the right side of the body that represents the masculine or solar energy

Pitta—one of the three doshas; the constitution of fire and water

Prakruti—one's inherent constitution, dosha, or nature established when one is conceived

Prana—life force, "breath"; the energy that is essential for life to exist

Ratricharya—Ayurveda's evening routine

Ritucharya—Ayurveda's seasonal routine

Ritusandhi—the transition or joint between the seasons

Samskara—a pattern, impression, or groove that is a result of conditioning; can be negative or positive

Shodhana—to purify or to cleanse

Svadhyaya—self-study

Swasthavritta—the code of conduct for preservation of health

Vaidya—physician or practitioner of Ayurveda

Vata—one of the three doshas; the constitution of ether and air

Vikruti—an imbalanced state of one's constitution or dosha

Yoga—Ayurveda's sister science; the practice of union between the mind, body, and self

Index

Acknowledgments

My nature is to resist help and figure things out on my own, as any pitta predominant person would do. However, by being in a community of like-minded and supportive people, I have learned that having help makes ideas, projects, relationships, and even one's health stronger. I am thankful to have received help from so many wonderful people in writing this book.

I will be forever grateful for my teachers and fellow classmates at Mount Madonna Institute, where I started my Ayurvedic journey. Their transmission of not only the knowledge of Ayurveda, but the essence, built my foundation and will always be a part of me.

To Cassandra Bodzak and my sisters in the book birthing club, your inspiration and support is what nurtured my dream of writing a book. You continue to inspire me daily.

To my literary agent, Steve Harris, and my editor, Jennifer Kurdyla, I'm thankful to have had your guidance, so that my ideas and experiences could be shaped into something more beautiful than I imagined.

To my Sage community, for always showing up, cheering me on, and laughing at my jokes. If everyone could have a supportive community like you, this world would be a much brighter place.

And finally, to my parents, Dan, and little Barry Allen. Your desire and willingness to help me fulfill my dreams never goes unnoticed.

About the Author

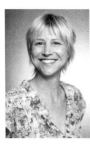 SARAH KUCERA, DC, CAP, has been championing healthy practices professionally for over a decade, and personally for her whole life. A licensed chiropractor, certified Ayurvedic practitioner, registered yoga teacher and yoga therapist, and entrepreneur, she is the founder of Sage, a healing arts center and herbal apothecary in Kansas City, Missouri, where she combines these methods to help others find well-being.

sarahkucera.com